Suc[...]t and Still

Finding joy and meaning through illness

Nin Mok

UpLit Press

© 2024 Nin Mok

Suddenly Silent and Still

First Edition, December 2024

Uplit Press

United Kingdom

https://uplitpress.co.uk/

Editing: UpLit Press

Cover Design: Nin Mok

Interior Formatting: UpLit Press

Suddenly Silent and Still is under copyright protection. No part of this book may be used or reproduced in any manner whatsoever without written permission except in the case of brief quotations embodied in critical articles and reviews. Printed in Adelaide, Australia. All rights reserved.

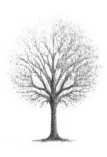

Join the Facebook Book Club

This group exists to give *Suddenly Silent and Still* readers an enhanced reading experience. It's a place to share thoughts, raise discussions and make friends while reading the book. Think of this group as a pop-up book club for those reading Suddenly Silent and Still.

facebook.com/groups/suddenlysilentandstill

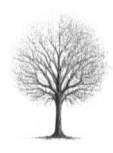

Prologue

There is nothing either good or bad, but thinking makes it so.
—*William Shakespeare, playwright and poet*

The pain of permanent separation and loss are quintessential human experiences. You may not have experienced that agony yet, but make no mistake—fate eventually pulls every name out of its hat.

I have no idea why I was certain my turn would come at the end of my life. I imagined myself being old and frail before discovering I had an incurable disease. I would then be afforded a moment of introspection before being shown the exit, like a happy-go-lucky partygoer who leaves when the music and fun are over. Never once did I imagine that I would have to stick around *after* the celebration for the long and arduous clean-up. Many of my beliefs, such as this one, turned out not to be true.

Another of my beliefs which was proven false was that there would be a warning before a life-changing disaster took place. Signs of an event that big were supposed to be hard to hide: the water receding into the ocean, wildlife fleeing in unprecedented numbers, people screaming; that kind of forewarning. Hiding a birthday cake from a child was a difficult enough feat, for goodness' sake. I was flabbergasted that I did not see a tragedy of such magnitude coming. There was no inkling of impending doom. It materialised out of the blue and left everlasting, disastrous consequences in its wake. Mother Nature was unsympathetic that I was in the middle of something important. She interrupted anyway.

I experienced gut-wrenching grief. My resilience was broken down, reducing me from a prowling lioness to a frightened little possum. I changed to the point that I could not recognise myself. Nothing remained the same, not my temperament, capabilities, confidence, or dreams. I had to work with this woman I no longer knew to reclaim my life. She was often too defeated or consumed by grief to even bother trying. The path of loss differs for everyone, but the feelings experienced are similar: fear, sadness, worthlessness, longing, anxiety, and panic.

Motivational speakers and self-help books were rife in claiming that "Happiness is a choice." I have come to recognise this messaging as toxic positivity. It was fine for people who were sick of their jobs or felt they were stuck in a rut. But for people like myself who were seriously grieving, who were most in need of happiness, the notion that happiness was a choice was condescending. It made me feel like I was grieving for too long, that I had become mopey and needed to snap out of it. It implied there was something wrong with me because I did not return to being happy after a few weeks of being sad.

Happiness was perhaps a choice if I was rushing home and got stuck in traffic or if the cork fell into my favourite wine bottle. Happiness was not a choice when I lost two major senses, hearing and balance, which snowballed into the loss of livelihood, connection, freedom, and myself. "Happiness is a choice" is insulting to people who have gone through serious grief. Try telling that to those who are terminally ill, or those who have waited nine months only to hold their stillborn baby, or those who have lost their spouse, limbs, mobility, minds, or entire fortunes.

Based on my lived experiences, I did not have a choice in how I reacted when tragedy blindsided and ambushed me. It felt similar to being swept away in a strong current. My emotions went wherever the turbulence took me. For a time, I was battered on boulders, grazed on sharp rocks, and swallowed a lot of water along the river of grief. It was a difficult and painful journey, but the river inevitably slowed at bends and eddies. At those moments, I had a choice: to scramble with all my might to the reedy banks and pull myself out or continue to drift with the current of sadness that would take me further away from a life I once knew and loved.

I never understood what my key strengths were until I was in my late thirties. They were not obvious nor easily translatable into a passion or career, such as painting, teaching, or some other talent. Not knowing what I was good at meant I didn't know what I wanted to be when I grew up. Long after I had grown up, I still didn't know. Then, a boss I much respected said to me, "I could drop you into any chaos and order would begin forming around you." He gestured concentric rings, a ripple that got bigger as it radiated outwards. Eureka. At the risk of sounding like a father searching for his kidnapped daughter, I had a very particular set of skills, skills that were innate and refined over a lengthy career. Those skills were bringing order to chaos.

I was employed for my skills under the guise of project management and executive leadership. My job was to rescue high-stakes projects, turn around problematic departments, and develop exemplary practices that were deployed organisation wide. After having fought fierce battles in the management arena, I can still state with conviction that my health tragedy was the most chaotic and complex situation I have ever dealt with. But, true to what my boss had observed, order began forming around my tragedy, and I grew to surpass it.

I couldn't choose to *be* happy, but I could choose to *seek* happiness. I could stoke the flames of life back from a traumatised ember into a roaring fire and hope that the essence of joy reignited. There were no guarantees that it would reunite me with happiness, but I had to try for myself and my family. People cannot live in mourning forever. To live in that state diminishes the flames of life, and when the light goes out, so does life. I would have died—at least metaphorically—from a broken heart if I carried the heavy sorrow for any longer than I did.

My A Gong's funeral was my first proper introduction to tragedy. I was twelve years old. Everyone was crying except my ama. She had been married to A Gong for over sixty years and still stood composed. A true matriarch, she comforted her children and grandchildren. Her hands were steady around our shoulders. "It will be okay," she told us with an unquivering voice. Both my grandparents had witnessed the Great Depression and World War II, yet their mental health was resolute. It was only after I experienced my tragedy that I realised why my grandparents possessed rock-solid resilience. Their experiences had set them up with an accurate understanding of reality. They never expected too much or too little of life, and their expectations were spot on. That gave them the armour to withstand life's cruel blows.

Suffering was the conjoined twin of painful experience. In hindsight, I suffered more than my pain. I suffered more than I needed to. My mental model of how the world worked had not adequately equipped me to deal with life's harsh realities, mostly because it was incorrect, comprised of too many rainbows and not enough clouds. Finding myself suddenly silent and still prompted me to ask the big questions. Why me? What is the meaning of this senseless suffering? Who am I now? And more importantly, how do I scramble back to the banks, and do I even want to? By asking the right questions, I gained the wisdom to turn my situation around. I updated my worldviews and put an end to my suffering, despite the pain persisting.

Ama set the bar high when she let go of A Gong with dignity and grace. In dealing with my significant loss, I too learned that nothing was outside my capability to endure. It was a matter of hanging in there long enough to let life do what it did best.

Given enough time, life finds a way. Many philosophers throughout history have explored this profound statement. Life, under any conditions, regardless of how harsh, will find a way to survive against all odds. My instincts wanted me to live. They wanted me to engage richly with my surroundings. Grief and circumstance could only contain my will for so long before life found a way. I was not shackled to my grief forever, and you won't be either. Given the opportunity to thrash around long enough in the deep end, everyone eventually learns to swim. Hang in there.

Support from my family was pivotal to my recovery, especially from Tom, my husband. He walked alongside me, ready to take over whenever I lacked the gumption to carry on. Without that safety net I would have lost my mind.

Besides taking care of me physically, Tom also supported my aspirations to write this book. His integrity is woven into every page. Tom could possibly be the only person in the world without a social media presence. He loathes performative platforms and what they stand for, the promotion of phony cultures that reward their users with validations for theatrics. Tom is a relationship-driven business executive whose success relies solely on his loyal customer' word of mouth, and he has never spent a dime on marketing and advertising. He is a walking oxymoron: the righteous businessman. That makes him the ideal gatekeeper of this memoir to ensure the story is told with sincerity and never veers off into exaggeration.

Our children were also pivotal in my recovery story. Jet and Jade were five and three when I got ill. They don't remember their healthy mother, the one who chased them through the parks, raced them to the car, and sang aloud, albeit out of tune. They just know this mother.

The one who struggled to make it through the day. Jet and Jade constantly needing my help and attention made my recovery more challenging, but at the same time, they made my recovery possible. Without their constant pull for me to join in their antics, I would have remained in bed indefinitely, absent of the will to go on. At times, I wished I was single and still living with my parents. It would have been nice to have them dote on me while I was grieving and ill. In hindsight, I am glad I had Jet and Jade around. Not only because they nudged me along in my recovery, but because I got to hear their little voices in stereo before all sounds flattened.

This memoir captures my journey in dealing with untimely and significant irreversible loss and the lessons I learnt along the way. It is a tale of how I chose life, applied the tools and wisdom that appeared before me, corrected my worldviews, and reinstated order from a state of traumatic chaos. Through this journey, I encountered many teachers of life. They resided in the wisdom of elderly people, children's untainted views, literature from thought leaders, uplifting stories of people who were in similar situations, and the merciless truths that nature tells. The immediate lesson was obvious: my situation had changed and so must I.

I wrote this memoir for both myself and others. Writing down thoughts is an effective way to extend memories. By putting ink to paper, the brain can begin to forget about it, be that the grocery list or a trauma. I prefer capturing and containing the terrifying memories that plague me between the pages of a book than having them continue to exist in my mind. Knowing that I have filed my story away in text, these troubled memories can fade. I will also leave my children with a tangible asset, a family blueprint, to get them through their own tough times ahead.

If you are going through a similar journey, I hope my discoveries can be of use to you. I apologise in advance for the heartbroken places this book will visit, but I promise, we will leave the dark tunnel behind together.

Chapter One

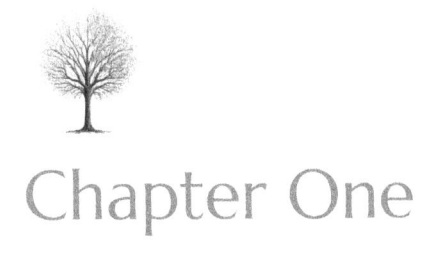

Chaos Before the Storm

Any idiot can face a crisis; it's this day-to-day living that wears you out.
—*Anton Chekhov, playwright and short story writer*

"For the tenth time, get out from underneath there!" Giggles and snorts continued as my two children turned the ironing board into a makeshift tent and monkey bars.

"It's raining," they cheered, reaching for the falling mist I sprayed onto the shirt for tomorrow's crucial meeting.

The department was finalising its annual budget, and I had to attend, fighting for every dollar for my office.

"The iron is hot. Play somewhere else." My warnings went unheeded, taking a backseat to the fun. They crawled around and in between my legs. The youngest, Jade, stopped to sit on my warm feet, briefly resting her back against my shins. Her simple gesture made me hyper-aware that I said "Not right now, Mummy is busy," more often than "Okay, I'll play with you." She sought a connection I struggled to give, overburdened with too many responsibilities and a packed schedule. I had no choice. *I'm a working mum doing her best.*

The ironing board bopped up and down under the weight of a swinging toddler, causing the iron to coast over the fabric like a jetski on the waves. I glared at my husband, Tom, his vacant eyes lost in space, his dust-speckled ankles marked by a day of laborious yard work. *Do something. Take the children.* I gave the kind of stare that burned, yet he remained zombified on the couch. He too appeared depleted and had no choice.

The long day had shortened my fuse. By early afternoon, I was fluent in frustration. After as much abuse as the ironing board could withstand, it crashed down onto the children, metal trusses clanking against their soft skulls. Laughter turned into wailing.

"This serves you two right!" I snapped, adrenaline rushing. Looking around for a place to put down my iron,

I realised this could have been much worse had I not been holding it. Yanking both children by their arms, I pulled them to their feet.

"Stop crying. Why are you crying when I already told you this would happen?" I scolded, cleaning up the cut on our son's forehead. Being taller than his sister, he bore the brunt of the accident. "You chose this," I ranted, losing my composure. Amidst his tears, the snorts became relentless, softening my heart. *Oh, Snortlepig.* I pulled him in close, holding back my own exhausted tears. I held his shaking body until the crying subsided. Tom and I endeared Jet with the nickname "Snortlepig", coined after a character in our favourite children's book, *Uno's Garden*, when he developed his distinctive tic.

Jet's tic had surfaced at three and worsened when he started primary school. Throughout the day, he would make loud snorting sounds, resembling an abrupt snore, the intensity and frequency varying with his emotions. People quickly suggested, or rather judged, that he was stressed. *Stressed about what? He was five years old.* Perhaps they saw something about our family that we were blind to.

The ironing board commotion broke Tom's trance, prompting him to get up and pursue the next chore. Startled into calmness, the children took over the empty couch and settled into a show. The brief respite allowed me to finish the ironing and Tom to start dinner.

Dinner was conversationless but far from commotionless. My attention was focused inward, planning meetings, deadlines and how to navigate office politics. Tom's mind was preoccupied with ensuring the livelihood of the growing number of families under his charge in his latest business venture. The children watched television while they ate but soon became restless. They left the table to run around, dipping back to replenish mouthfuls before taking off again. Food crumbs scattered throughout the house where they ran. Neither one of us summoned them back to the table. There was no energy left for this battle.

I trudged into the kitchen to prepare tomorrow's lunches while Tom washed up at a manic speed, willing the day to end.

"There are ten thousand ten-minute chores to do," I muttered, cutting grapes in half to prevent choking hazards. "It never ends."

"I don't do anything I enjoy anymore," Tom agreed, sighing. "This arrangement is unsustainable."

Meanwhile, Jet and Jade raided the treat-filled pantry to their heart's content. I didn't mind. Time-pressed, I took every shortcut to their smiles, compensating them with too many treats, new toys, and other gimmicks. It distracted them from noticing I was not around enough and helped me not feel guilty about it. I ran their bath with extra bubbles. *This outrageous foam mountain should do the trick*, I thought, turning off the tap and leaving them to bathe themselves. They squealed with delight, cleaning each other with squirt guns.

By the time the children were bathed and tucked into bed, Tom and I found one another again, collapsed on the couch; shells of our former selves with soulless eyes. We reached for each other's hands, our fingers intertwining tightly. It was less of a romantic gesture and more us desperately clinging to one another with whatever our weary bodies had left.

"Let's watch something. Anything you want, darling," Tom said, tucking a loose strand of hair behind my ear. The clock permitted a short sitcom before signalling bedtime.

The remote sat a few feet from us with no takers. Fatigued, we let the television dictate its own program. A salesman on the screen transformed a mop into a duster and a broom, demonstrating its effectiveness. His sales pitch washed over us.

Emotionally spent, with a heavy mind and a tired body, I crossed the bedroom doorway, imagining the victory ribbon falling away around my waist. Scraping through with no reserves left, I wondered whether I should be so lucky tomorrow. Every day was touch and go.

The morning alarm at our house triggered the same chaos as a siren in a fire station day room. All hands and feet had to move if everyone was to reach their destination on time.

"Cereal again?" Jet protested, scrunching his face in disgust.

"It looks like dog biscuits," Jade added, mirroring her brother's sentiment.

"Then add milk," I ordered. Cold cereal in winter was all a hectic family could afford. Memories of my childhood, with warm savoury congee and dumpling soups for breakfast flashed through my mind, compounding my guilt. *Times are different now*, I rationalised.

Jet's school was on the way to Tom's work, making him responsible for school drop-offs and pickups. I had no relationship with Jet's teachers, nor had I seen the classroom projects he boasted about. After school, Jet claimed the boardroom in Tom's office, babysat with snacks and unlimited screen time. He even joined the occasional meeting as an uninvited guest. Every day, Tom brought our son to work, compromising his professional environment. Tom refused to place Jet in after-school care and showed his love through proximity. Daddy, though unreachable, was just next door, separated by a wall. Jet loved it.

Following a similar logic, I managed Jade's childcare arrangements. Our family carer was located on my commute to work. Tom missed witnessing her forming her first friendships and many other milestones. We were parenting in halves.

"Mummy, can you please pick me up earlier today?" Jade pleaded. "I'm always the last kid left."

"I'll see what I can do."

We both knew that meant "no". I smiled, squeezing her tight, breathing in her warmth and scent, not wanting to let go. Jade's expression remained crestfallen, adding another straw to my mother's guilt, ever closer to its breaking point.

Chapter Two

Befallen

There is no despair so absolute as that which comes with the first moments of our darkest hours.
—*Mary Ann Evans, novelist*

Tragedies love to begin their day unassumingly. I was working from the comfort of home, overlooking our pristine vegetable garden. Shirt pressed, hair straightened, but still in sweatpants, I began my first Skype meeting of the day. We had barely covered the agenda when blaring ringing in my ears interrupted me, similar to how a grenade goes off near an unsuspecting soldier. I assumed my headset was faulty and persevered to the end of the meeting.

After exiting Skype, I removed my headset and was surprised to hear the ringing continue. Blocking my ears with my hands did nothing to lower the volume. I dug around in my ear canals, as if to perform a factory reset on my hearing, and realised the rustling sound could only be heard in my right ear. I wasn't worried. I remembered walking out of countless concerts in my twenties with ears ringing so loud that my friends and I had to shout at one another to converse. The ringing always subsided the next day. *Surely the same will happen here. The volume on my headset must have been set too loud.*

Soon after, I felt lightheaded. Graced with a few seconds to do so, I staggered to my bed. The woozy feeling escalated, now akin to being uncaremoniously kicked out of an aeroplane without a parachute, spinning violently out of control and falling to my death. I screamed in panic and clawed at the bed sheets. I clung on desperately until the room became still and the walls met at the corners once again.

I soon realised any movement would trigger violent vertigo, so I laid motionless. Freezing cold, I could not manoeuvre my way under the covers. Thank goodness I was in sweatpants. Little did I know that these sweatpants that were labouring to keep me warm against winter's bite would later become my undoing. I lay there thinking this was simply a case of low electrolytes or iron levels. I had been working too hard and just needed a vitamin boost. Several hours passed before I heard keys jingling, signalling my husband's return home from work. Finally, Tom could call an ambulance.

The tornado in my mind was relentless, exacerbated by the entire transition from my house to the emergency department and finally to a ward. The Australian hospital system was under enormous strain, and the move became an eleven-hour exercise. I vomited myself to exhaustion from motion sickness whilst a nurse took control of my head because I'd lost the ability to discern which direction was skyward. Another nurse administered a cocktail of chemicals intravenously to stabilise my world but to nil effect. It did, however, reframe my reaction. I was no longer in a state of panic, free falling to my death. I was now calm, trippy, and twirling out into space.

No longer troubled by my dizziness, other sensations rose to the forefront. The dam was cracking.

"You're going to have to go sometime. Can't keep it in forever, love," said the nurse with a knowing smile as she walked off with the bedpan I had declined. It had been nearly ten hours since I last emptied my bladder, but I was not prepared for her to flush my dignity down the toilet just yet. Perhaps I could hold on a little while longer until I was steady enough to make my way to the restroom. That had been my plan for several hours, and

I had now pushed well beyond the limits of holding it. Having my bottom wiped pre-dated my earliest memory, and I was not about to create a fresh imprint of it that could be recalled on demand going forward. The pain was excruciating. I imagined what would happen if my bladder burst, and began assessing what my dignity was worth. I was playing a game of chicken with Mother Nature, and she was about to swerve my stubbornness off the road.

I rang the bell to call the nurse back in. Feeling awkward, I insisted that Tom assist me instead of her. "Suit yourself," she said, placing the bedpan at the end of my bed. My bladder must have been horrifically numb from my failings to service it since it took twenty minutes to start the trickle.

An uncomfortable first-date feeling occurred between Tom and me, concerned about what the other was thinking but not saying. He broke the tension by being jovial. "Before we had children, this may have been a big deal. But I've changed the kids' nappies so often that this has become a non-event. Your bum is just bigger," he teased. And just like a muscle can tear and repair to become stronger from a strenuous workout at the gym, the invisible boundaries of polite formalities within our marriage broke down and were redefined, strengthening our unity.

Discomfort, it appeared, followed a hierarchy of needs. The vertigo subsided now that I was no longer in transit and could lie statue still, and my bladder pains had also been alleviated. My focus quickly turned to how sweaty I felt. My face felt flushed, and my palms were clammy. I was not complying with the patient's uniform, which was essentially a reversed kimono made from wafer-thin, breathable blue cloth with two strings at the back that held everything together. The garment was clearly designed with easy access in mind. The hospital's thermostat was set to summer to accommodate this free-flowing attire, and I was inappropriately dressed for the occasion, having come in from the winter weather outside. My pullover business shirt with a collar had no buttons to undo that could relieve me from the heat. My once cosy sweatpants now betrayed me. Changing clothes was out of the question. Any movement felt like I was in a washing machine, and I did not want to start the throwing-up cycle all over again. I would remain in this sweltering outfit for the next three days.

"Fresh-out-of-the-oven warm blankets, anyone?" a nurse asked, making her rounds.

A face I didn't recognise drew back the curtains, entering my cramped quarters. There must have been a shift change. "I'm here to take your blood pressure," she said as she wrapped a cuff around my arm. "Now please sit up."

"I can't. I have vertigo and will vomit again," I explained.

"Please sit up. We need to work out if your vertigo is blood-pressure related. I'll take your blood pressure once you're sitting and then once more when you're standing," she said. *Standing? She must be out of her mind*, I thought.

"I can't move my head by a centimetre. How am I going to sit up? No, I can't," I protested.

"You have to," she ordered like one would tell a child to finish their vegetables. Unconvinced by my condition, she slid her arm underneath my back and attempted to raise me into a sitting position. I was barely above the pillow when the room accelerated, and I vomited all over myself. My stomach was out of content, so the cleanup was minimal for her, to my vengeful disdain. She laid me back down while I dry retched. "Okay, we'll leave it for now," she said and left in a manner as entitled as her demands. No apology. No sympathy. I never saw her again. She must have palmed me off to her colleague after that awkward exchange.

The registrar in charge ordered an ECG and an MRI. "Someone will come and collect you soon," he said.

I had never seen Tom look so sad as he stood bedside. He had not left me even to get a drink of water or a much-needed coffee. It had been eight hours since he found me lying debilitated.

"Are you worried?" I asked.

"Vertigo meds didn't work. Now they're ordering an ECG to check your heart and an MRI to check your brain.

Yes, I'm worried. I don't like where this is heading," he replied.

Tom worked in the clinical informatics space, where information technology is used to optimise the management of healthcare data to improve patient care, enhance clinical workflows, and advance medical research. He had analysed countless cases that ended in mortality, making him well-versed in these scenarios and statistics. How my situation was unfolding filled his heart with dread as he fixated on the possibility of a stroke, brain tumour, or brain bleed. I was not worried in the slightest because fear of when the spinning would start again consumed my mind. I was in survival mode. When chased by a tiger, you don't look to the next month or even the next day. I was busy running, not planning my potential funeral.

The ECG was straightforward, taking a few minutes to complete. Heart monitoring pads were stuck in strategic positions around my chest, and beats were charted on the screen. Thankfully, they didn't need me to move to capture the squiggles.

An orderly showed up soon after to transport me to my MRI. "Please don't move her too much. She has vertigo," Tom said with his hand resting on my bed, signalling I was not to be taken until there was an understanding between him and the orderly. After the blood pressure debacle with that heartless nurse, he wasn't keen on another round of insensitivity. The orderly gave a nod of acknowledgement, and Tom removed his hand from my bed, green-lighting him to take me.

The sterile-white MRI room's ceiling was tiled with LCD screens. Together, the screens displayed seamless footage of long, vibrant grass swaying in a gentle breeze under clear blue skies. Colourful wildflowers dotted the picturesque meadow. Day spa music played from the speakers mounted around the room. The overcompensation of serenity raised my suspicion. I felt like a cow following a rattling tin of feed onto the slaughter truck.

The Grand Canyon chasm between where I lay and the MRI table seemed impossible to traverse. My look gave it away. "We'll make it work," said the lady who would be conducting my MRI. She wheeled my bed parallel to the table and lowered it to match its height.

"I can't move at all," I warned her, panicking, pointing to the vomit bag beside me. "I have vertigo and I'll throw up." She gave a reassuring smile and flattened my bed railings. Using a reverse tablecloth trick, she pulled my bedsheet slowly across onto the MRI table, taking with it all the contents and myself. I hardly had to move.

She placed a safety button in my left hand and explained it was a tap-out button. She then put the vomit bag in my other hand, just in case. I got the hint. The impressive machine looked like it came from the future and must have cost a fortune. I didn't want to be the person who threw up in it. She placed headphones on me and left the room. The spa music streamed directly into my hearing ear. "Are you ready?" Her voice interrupted the tranquil melody. "We're about to start. Make sure you stay perfectly still and don't move an inch," she instructed. I smirked at the irony.

The noisy machine powered up, and I was transitioned into its dark tunnel. I had forgotten to ask if I could keep my eyes open and whether these death rays would blind me. I closed my eyes as a precaution. Loud banging occurred in a rhythmic series as panels fired up, drowning out the soothing music. The space warmed up. I was already hot and sweaty; now I was baking in a tiny oven. Even with my eyes closed, I felt claustrophobic. Air felt different in the small space. There was nothing natural about this experience, hence the rattling feed tin to lure me in. I persevered until it was over.

The registrar examined my ECG and MRI results. "All looks normal," he said, ruling out stroke and brain tumour as probable causes, even though, as he explained, their presentations were similar to what I was displaying. Tom breathed a sigh of relief. The registrar diagnosed me with labyrinthitis, a fanciful way of saying I had a common cold that had gone rogue. I was asymptomatic and did not recall a single sniffle or even a scratchy throat. The alleged virus snuck its way into my inner ear, destroying the hearing and balance nerves that neighboured one another. This meant

I was now deaf in my left ear, and my brain could no longer interpret any motion cues.

My brain compensated for the silence in my left ear by courteously simulating an unbearable high-pitched ringing sound. Doctors call this phenomenon tinnitus. The ringing was an unwelcome alarm clock in my head with no off button. I immediately thought of the iconic scene from *Dumb and Dumber* where Lloyd turns to his friends in the van and asks, "Want to hear the most annoying sound in the world?" He then screams within the small confinement of their vehicle. One of his friends blows a gasket after five seconds, and yet I was supposed to be okay with hearing this sound for the rest of my life?

My condition was now stable, and the emergency room doctor had given us his best guess diagnosis. I was no longer a high-risk patient and could finally be transferred to my permanent ward.

"You have no reason to watch over me. You better go home. It's six in the morning," I said.

"I'm not leaving," Tom insisted.

"Just go. I'll be okay," I reassured him. "I'll see you tomorrow. Get some sleep. Our kids need a parent, and my mum could use a break."

I did not sleep a wink that night, too afraid that I would move in my sleep and go into a spin. Daylight was already bleeding through the blinds by the time I nodded off for a moment, not daring to sleep long enough to change positions.

The next few days in the hospital were spent no differently than if I had been paralysed. I remained in bed, being spoon-fed, drinking through a bent straw, and needing assistance with a bedpan. At home, I wiped little bottoms, but here in the hospital, I was the big baby. They even placed a bib on me at mealtimes. Thank goodness they didn't do the aeroplane to feed me. My dignity couldn't handle much more assault.

My limbs felt like they were attached to my head by puppet strings. I could not lift them without my ears firing false signals to my brain, sending me into a traumatising spin. Every bone and muscle in my body ached, longing for movement. I wiggled my fingers and toes to get some relief.

"Just hang in there a while longer. Twenty-four hours is hardly long in the big scheme of things," scoffed the warden of a doctor who was doing the morning rounds. She managed to provide some comforting words, reassuring me that the brain was quite clever. In a few days, it would realise something was amiss, deducing that it was improbable for me to be spinning at the rate of an audacious fairground ride for this long. My brain would then begin to rewire and reinterpret these broken signals, affording me some relief. She tempered my expectations by cautioning that this was going to be a sloth of a process. My need for productivity and progress made me an impatient patient, and she understood this was going to be a frustrating recovery process for me.

Tom cleared his calendar that week to be with me in the hospital. He visited during work hours while the children maintained their childcare routine. We had not been alone for such an extended period since before our eldest, Jet, arrived five years ago. Amidst the health chaos, Tom and I began to rediscover each other after losing one another to the grind of busy careers and taking care of our children. We began reconnecting. That week, despite our circumstance, we smiled, giggled, bantered, locked eyes, shared food, and explored hypothetical scenarios like new lovers. Magic was blooming.

"The military really needs to tap into this. Imagine being able to induce vertigo during interrogations. Forget waterboarding," Tom said after observing my situation.

"The toughest terrorists would crack within the hour," I replied.

We balanced the whimsical energy in the room with long stretches of comfortable silence. After all, we weren't new lovers. Quiet or chatty, we delighted in each other's company, appreciating this rare opportunity. What we didn't appreciate was the seriousness of our predicament. It felt too surreal to be true. We both believed I would heal and that normality would return soon enough.

Our reconnection trivialised lingering disputes, rendering them as petty. We wiped our resentment slates clean that week and forgave each other's shortcomings in our marriage. We were grateful to still have one another. "I see you," I said to Tom whilst forehead to forehead. He felt it too. "Labyrinthitis saves marriages," became Tom's mantra. Not that our marriage needed any real saving. Just as pressure creates diamonds, hardship forges strong bonds. Our love ran deep because we shared many positives, including a home and children. Our love now ran deeper still because we shared adversity and were adamant to see it through together. The helper felt useful and heroic, and the person being helped felt loved and grateful. It was the perfect win-win exchange.

An ear, nose, and throat specialist (ENT) entered my room, pushing a tray of bits and bobs. She held a silver metal horseshoe implement a couple of inches away from my broken ear and struck it with a metal rod.

"Nothing," I replied. I could not hear a thing. She pressed the horseshoe to my skull right behind my ear and whacked it again. The vibrations bypassed my eardrum and went straight to my hearing nerves. Again, I could not hear a thing. She concluded that my hearing nerves were either inflamed or dead. To rescue these audio nerves, she prescribed high-dose oral steroids that I would take for two months, hoping they would reduce the inflammation.

"Will I be able to hear again?" I blurted, even though I was not ready to hear the answer.

"There is a thirty per cent chance you will recover hearing on your own, a thirty per cent chance that you will recover hearing with treatment, and a thirty per cent chance you will not recover your hearing at all," she replied, void of emotion.

Tom, a man who enjoyed his cold beers and weekend punting, was comfortable with those odds. "You will hear again, love," he said with confidence.

I thought, *What about the last ten per cent? Does the virus spread to other nerves? Do I go deaf in both ears?* It turned out that sums didn't need to add up in medicine, which was a bit of a worry.

Five days later, I could stand, and even shuffle my feet inch by inch, aided by a framed walker and a nurse. I felt like I was in a small dinghy on treacherous seas rather than on tiled floors that obeyed gravity. The moment I made it to the restroom a few meters away without falling, unassisted by human help, I declared that I was going home.

My three- and five-year-olds were waiting impatiently for their mum to return. They could not visit because of Covid restrictions. My heart ached because I was not providing the cuddles and kisses they were yearning for. Since they were born, I had not missed one tuck-in, and now I had missed seven. I requested to leave the hospital because being a mum trumped being a patient. Reluctantly, the hospital discharged me. They made it clear to Tom that returning home did not mean returning to home duties; it was still bedrest and operating strictly under hospital conditions. He agreed.

The acute phase had ended. I cannot recall my feelings during that week with clarity, most likely because there were none. I was simply thinking of myself as a tourist in this tragedy, soon to return to my typical day of commuting to work and picking up groceries on the way home. This mindset made me a compliant patient, willingly wheeled from one medical activity to the next on the diagnostic obstacle course. Upon being discharged from the hospital with a walker, the reins were handed over to the rehabilitation team. There were a few more sights for this tourist to see yet, and soon I would be home, truly home, fully hearing, and well-balanced. Or so I thought.

Chapter Three

Race Against Time

The harder the conflict, the more glorious the triumph. What we obtain too cheap, we esteem too lightly; it is dearness only that gives everything its value.
—*Thomas Paine, political philosopher*

I was one of the lucky six who drew the long straw to take part in the hospital's trial program and was granted access to their new hyperbaric chamber. I put on the provided jumpsuit and made my way to the white container-like construction that stood in the centre of an expansive room. The inside resembled a rocket ship. The nurse ushered me into a plush recliner, but I could not find comfort. Unfamiliarity filled me with anticipation.

The nurse lowered a domed helmet over my head that fit snugly around my neck. The helmet had a clear screen I could see through. Tubes dangled from its top, making their way to the walls. A small smile broke through at how novel it felt, like I was an astronaut about to launch into space. The tiny room was just big enough to fit six of these setups, three on each side, with a narrow aisle through the middle. A nurse stood stationed at the front, just in case. *Just in case of what, exactly?*

My fellow voyagers for the day consisted of five gentlemen, upwards of their mid-seventies. I was the Smurfette who held back the average age within the chamber. The democratic system broke down under such narrow and polarising demographics, and a Western cowboy movie from the sixties was voted in for us to view on the mounted television screen.

The nurse wandered down the aisle, flicking on the switches above our heads one by one. Oxygen flowed liberally into our masks, three times the concentration we usually breathe. Then the cabin pressurisation process began, equivalent to descending fourteen meters under the sea. I automatically reached to pinch my nose and pop my ears, but they were locked away behind my helmet. I opened my mouth wide as if to yawn, allowing me to equalise the changing pressure as we descended.

I expected pure oxygen in high concentration to feel like a stroll in an ancient forest. Instead, it felt like sitting in a stuffy wardrobe. The smell of the clear plastic a couple of inches from my face was overpowering. I was a claustrophobic Russian doll, my head enclosed in a helmet whilst I was sitting in a tiny chamber, denied of windows. The tiny space felt even smaller without outside views, and the air I was breathing in felt foreign. I tried to remain calm, fighting against primitive instincts to seek the air I was used to.

I was not accustomed to downtime, and two hours in the chamber felt like four. As a mum of two energetic young children who also maintained a demanding career, I was unfamiliar with watching movies for fun. This Western felt like the longest movie ever produced.

I had to return the next day at the crack of dawn. These hyperbaric chamber sessions were to occur over twenty consecutive days, during which the doctor would evaluate me for any improvements before deciding whether to continue with further sessions. The idea of the hyperbaric chamber was to flood the body with high levels of oxygen, supercharging the healing process. I was told I had a small window of opportunity for my hearing to return, that most of the recovery would happen in the first two weeks, and that after three months, whatever was lost would be gone forever. I was now at the start of week three. It was a race against time to recover my hearing. The doctor believed the hyperbaric chamber to be a long shot, but she was willing to give it a try. Considering that each session cost north of one thousand dollars, and I was receiving the treatment for free, I was prepared to do my part, even if it meant enduring a daily dose of *The Good, The Bad and The Ugly* or its equivalent.

After a week in the chamber with no recovery to my hearing, I decided it would only be prudent to do my due diligence. We reached out to all our medical contacts, family, friends, and associates. Three independent recommendations came back for the best ENT in the city, who had a long waitlist. We pulled strings and cashed in favours, allowing me to see him that afternoon.

We were called into his examination room. My explanation of "I cannot hear anything" was not convincing enough. His audiologist conducted a hearing test like the one I had recently undertaken at the hospital, and this reconfirmed the results—my left ear was dead. He asked me what had happened. Fully aware of how fiercely specialists guarded their time, I began to summarise my story.

Before I could finish, he cut me off mid-sentence with a stern monotone voice, reminiscent of God laying down the commandments. "Your hearing is gone! It's not coming back! When your feelings settle, make another appointment to discuss options. As for your balance, don't expect to be riding bikes ever again."

My eyes welled up with tears as this sentence was handed to me without the possibility of appeal. I turned to Tom for comfort, only to see his eyes narrowed and fixated on the specialist, like a lion stalking its prey.

Dr. Ellen Langer, a renowned Harvard psychologist, states in an interview that "Medical science like all science can only give us probabilities." She explains how medical journals present probabilities as absolutes and criticizes doctors who deliver a diagnosis in such definitive terms. Langer believes it to be detrimental for patients to receive such a diagnosis because it impairs the brain-body connection in the healing process. Whatever the mind believes, the body has a better chance of becoming. An absolute diagnosis is therefore not only false, but also unhelpful.

Tom knew this from his day job.

The ENT specialist asked Tom if he had any questions. Tom probed aggressively at what he felt to be an unjustified level of resoluteness. The specialist seemed unaccustomed to being challenged, and Tom's line of questioning resulted in a heated exchange. The atmosphere was so tense it snapped me out of my sorrows.

On the walk back to the car park, he said, "I don't care what happens. We are not going back to see that incompetent, arrogant asshole again!"

This translated to "My heart is broken for you, my darling" after witnessing the doctor tersely deliver my verdict and my subsequent devastation. I was not the only one suffering in this tragedy; Tom was hurting too.

Between the hyperbaric chamber, the audiologist, the neurophysiotherapist, and the ENT specialist, I returned to the hospital daily. On certain days, I made multiple appearances. I could not drive myself, having the coordination of an alcoholic on payday, so chauffeuring me to and from my rehabilitation schedule became a full-time job for Tom, who already had a full-time job. Tragedy, it seemed, was a team sport.

Tom would find a quiet corner in a waiting room to set up his nomadic office, taking meetings while "Attention! Code blue!" blasted on the intercom. At home, he held the fort, buying groceries, cooking, cleaning, bathing the kids, and reading bedtime stories. All the while, I was propped up in bed, wedged in place with a pile of pillows as if I had no skeleton. There was nothing I could do but helplessly watch as the pressure-cooker situation built up day by day in our home. Tom loathed asking for help and carried the weight entirely on his shoulders. He felt it was solely his responsibility to take care of his family.

Concurrent with the daily hyperbaric chamber sessions, I received weekly intratympanic steroid injections. The doctor inserted a long needle containing steroids into my eardrums, depositing the liquid straight to the middle ear, as near as possible to ground zero. She hoped the steroids would reduce inflammation of the fine hair-like nerves that were responsible for hearing—or, in my case, not hearing.

I was instructed to hold completely still while the needle penetrated my eardrum. I recalled cleaning my ears too deeply once with a cotton bud and how that had felt. Sitting mannequin-still through this seemed an impossible request. The doctor first injected local anaesthetic close to my eardrum on the wall of my ear canal to assist with the impending pain. The anaesthetic trickled down the back of my throat, burning it with great discomfort and impeding my ability to swallow. Just another odd sensation to add to the growing list. Finally, the cold liquid steroid was delivered deep into my ear, triggering vertigo. I lay still, my arms wrapped around my knees.

"See you again next week," said the specialist lackadaisically after my vertigo subsided.

Sorry, I thought, *but I would need to be dragged back here by a herd of elephants for the second injection to happen*. I am convinced people only benchmark against labour pains because they have never had a needle go through their eardrum before. I have now done both and would prefer to give birth to several more children.

At home that night, I was a defeated mess. I never wanted to go through that again, and knowing that I would have to do so in seven days left me unsettled.

Standing together in the middle of our kitchen, Tom pulled me in and held me close with my bad ear to his chest, as if to protect it from any more harm. I expected to hear his heartbeat as I usually did. Instead, there was total silence, as if I was holding a corpse. That was truly the last straw. The tension that had built up from spending the day as a lab rat broke loose, and tears streamed uncontrollably down my face.

"I want the first sound I hear to be your heartbeat, my love," I cried.

I managed to reset my emotions overnight and regained enough composure to attend my rehabilitation the following morning. Within the hyperbaric chamber, communication with my fellow patients had progressed from polite nods and awkward smiles into small talk. By the tenth session, it matured into deep conversations about shared pains and fears. The gentleman behind me extended his friendship by sharing his story. He had prostate cancer. He underwent brachytherapy, a procedure that inserted permanent radioactive metal seeds into his prostate organ, slowly releasing low-dose radiation. These seeds were causing him to feel sick but could not be easily removed. Worse, the brachytherapy did not end up being effective in treating his cancer, and he was now stuck with them forever releasing radiation into his body. The next treatment he underwent was a prostatectomy, a surgery to remove the cancerous part of his prostate. He sustained rectal injuries as a complication from the procedure, and though the risks were minimal, he became a statistic.

His injuries were not healing on their own, securing him a seat in the hyperbaric chamber. Breathing concentrated oxygen was his last hope before he would need to have a tube installed in his stomach with a colostomy bag at the other end. He would need to carry and manage this bag for the rest of his life. Not only would this be a significant habit change from merely having to flush, but his invisible illness would become visible. He'd had thirty sessions in the chamber so far with no improvements. His prospects looked grim. He laid out his regrets candidly. In hindsight, he would have been happier to live with the slow-growing cancer that would have claimed his life in ten years or more. He would have gracefully transitioned into his eighties by then, having lived a quality life, and would have been content to call it quits. Instead, he would now spend his last decade fussing around with faeces.

He explained that doctors were more knowledgeable about diseases than their patients, however, their motivations differed from their patients'. Doctors wanted to conquer diseases at all costs, whereas patients wanted to live their best life possible. These two differing objectives were at odds with one another, especially in his case. He'd trusted the medical system, and it let him down. He encouraged me to research as much as possible and to advocate for my health. Only I had the full picture of how I felt, what I wanted to achieve, and what I would sacrifice for it.

I felt slightly happier hearing his story, not because he was suffering, but because I was not alone or being singled out by the universe. Guilt suddenly washed over me. I must be a terrible person to take any joy from a story like this.

As these sessions rolled on, my taste in movies broadened, judging by my feeling of disappointment when I could not finish one of these Western or wartime movies. I would watch them attentively and always be robbed of the ending. After the nurse gave her introductory speech about the exits being here and there, the remaining duration in the chamber was just shy of a movie length. I had to imagine the last ten minutes, and I am certain cowboys have never been more sentimental than they were in my version of the endings.

The men were busy discussing the would-be conclusion to the latest movie when a minor miracle happened. I could hear a representation of them through my dead ear, not speaking, but mumbling incomprehensibly. It sounded like they were speaking in a library with their lips sewn together. I rushed out as fast as my walker could take me to tell Tom the exciting news. I gave him a celebratory hug, placing my bad ear against his chest.

Ba-boom, ba-boom! Sure enough, I could hear his heart beating again.

I spent the day biting down my nails. I had my hearing assessment that afternoon, and the improvements made, albeit minor, meant that the ENT specialist would insist on a second intratympanic steroid injection. I knew what to expect this time, and it was far worse than what I had imagined the first time around. I felt my limbs stiffen. My brain had to override all natural inclinations to flee. My mind exited the room, leaving my emotionless shell of a body to get the job done. An appointment was made for the third injection the next week, should I keep showing improvements in my hearing. An internal conflict developed. The fighter in me wanted to keep healing, and the little girl in me wanted progress to stagnate so I never had to endure these god-awful injections ever again.

The next morning, a relatively young man hobbled into the chamber, aided by a pair of crutches, replacing the senior gentleman who had been seated in the back row. I never got to know the gentleman who left, for no reason other than the recliner that divided us. I spared a quiet thought to wish him well on his journey. Being in the chamber meant he had a tough battle that he needed to win. We all did. The newcomer said a quick "Hello" and proceeded to his station before striking up a conversation, which violated the first-session protocol of polite nods only. "What are you all in for?" he asked, directing the question at everyone with enthusiasm.

I noticed his foot was wrapped tightly in bandages that seeped crimson. I tried hard to avert my gaze. He shared that he was a type two diabetic, and that poor wound healing was part of the insidious package. He had stubbed his toe on his bed several weeks before, causing severe inflammation and swelling that would not resolve on its own. Most of us would have simply said "Ouch" and been able to move on. He, on the other hand, had to have several toes amputated. Upon that revelation, I immediately noticed that he was also missing digits on both hands. He exuded the energy of a motivational speaker, cheery and upbeat despite what he was going through. I was keen to unlock the mystery of his smile.

It turned out that he had been a diabetic since he was a child and had been managing the condition throughout most of his life. Like a skilled sailor adept at navigating rough seas, he was proficient at dealing with misfortunes. Amputation was just the tip of the iceberg. People with type two diabetes are prone to kidney diseases because their kidneys must work overtime to remove excess glucose from their blood. His kidneys had long ago given up, and the hospital matched him with a donor kidney. The organ transplant was a success, and he could live to fight another day. He learnt how to brace himself for these hits when they came, and they kept coming for him. Dealing with misfortune appeared to be like any other skill, be it painting or swimming. With practice, he became good at it. I could too.

After he finished sharing his story, my eyes felt heavy, and my blinks were getting slower. Two hours in the chamber was a long time to be doing nothing. I began dozing off, and my head dropped. I awoke in a state of panic from the sensation of simultaneously falling and rapidly spinning. "Help me, somebody help me!" I screamed, trying not to slide off the chair. In the split second I came out of sleep, I did not know where I was. I scrambled to find reality. Maybe I was in space, and a meteorite had just hit my ship. That would explain the astronaut suit and why I was spinning out of control.

The nurse rushed to my aid, freeing me from my helmet. "You are all right; you have vertigo. Hold still," she instructed. She decided I would not be resuming my session. Still in a state of distress, I pleaded with her to continue my therapy. I did not want to miss my shot at getting back my hearing. She did not change her mind. It was an expensive price to pay for dozing off.

No drama in the chamber could match that of the intratympanic steroid injections, which had come around again. I made myself cosy in the furthest corner of the waiting room. The ENT specialist was running over an hour late. As far as I was concerned, the later the better. I was in no rush to get my third injection.

Eventually, I was called in. My hearing test showed no improvements from the previous week. People still sounded like the hushed version of hooded Kenny from *South Park*. I was sad to learn that I had made no improvements, but this was balanced out by the ENT specialist declaring a third injection would not be required. These injections were traumatic for patients, and unless there was clear evidence of improvements, the hospital would not authorise further injections. I breathed a sigh of relief.

My intensive rehabilitation was almost finished. There were no more injections to be had and only one more hyperbaric chamber session to complete.

"Today is my last day in the chamber, guys," I announced on entry.

I felt a bit deflated. I was parting with my newfound friends. We had bonded over our vulnerabilities, each willingly trading intimate stories. In my other world, free of afflictions, friends wouldn't even share selfies taken without a filter, and here I was amongst strangers, each of us contributing to our deep conversations, void of pretentiousness. The genuine side of humanity was the single rose on the thorny stem of tragedy. I was grateful to have experienced true heartfelt connections.

"Go on, then! You can pick the movie today," offered the cowboys. Flicking through the listings, I was tempted to repay them with *Clueless* or *Legally Blonde*. That would surely change the energy in the room. However, I could not be happy unless everyone was happy.

"*Shawshank Redemption*, please," I requested.

The hospital advised me that they had come to the end of the line in terms of the treatments they could offer for my hearing. The ENT specialist informed me that recovery of any hearing was unlikely from this point on. It had been six weeks since the onset of my profound hearing loss, and the statistics were no longer in my favour. The hospital wanted to arrange a professional counsellor to help me process my feelings. Unless the psychologist could make me hear again, I was not interested. Pragmatic me was capable of crying on my own, thank you. For my consolation prize, the ENT specialist explained that my balance would continue to improve and that rehabilitation with a neurophysiotherapist could now begin.

I felt like I had been ejected from a fighter jet. Everything had happened so fast, and just like that, it had come to an abrupt stop without a proper landing. The hospital's automatic double doors parted. Stepping out into the daylight, I felt naked, like a baby bird prematurely forced out of its nest to fend for itself. How could I possibly return home and carry on as if nothing had happened?

Chapter Four

Bargaining with the Universe

Have patience with everything that remains unsolved in your heart. Try to love the questions themselves, like locked rooms and the books written in a foreign language. Do not now look for the answers. They cannot now be given to you because you could not live them. It is a question of experiencing everything. At present you need to live the question. Perhaps you will gradually, without even noticing it, find yourself experiencing the answer some distant day.
—*Rainer Maria Rilke, poet and novelist*

"Do you need anything?" Tom asked, about to head off to work, as he kissed me goodbye on my forehead.

"Nope. I'm securely wedged into place," I replied.

A book would have been nice, but blurred vision and dizziness denied me the pleasure of reading. He left the room where I sat propped up in bed, my position no different from yesterday. After the windowless hospital and the sterile hyperbaric chamber, I was grateful to be back home, sitting in my bed, with a view. The bedroom window overlooked the walk-in chicken coop that Tom had designed and built. An ordinary-looking grey pigeon flew to perch on its wooden frame, pacing back and forth to survey the lands below. It swooped down to the coop floor, littered with chicken feed, and helped itself to the seed buffet. When it reemerged back on top of the frame, our staring contest began.

Pigeons live for around ten years, I thought, *and humans, eighty*. That meant one hour of my time was equivalent to eight of his. Lifespan was in my favour, and victory was assuredly mine. Three hours went by. I did not move, only to be matched by this stubborn pigeon. What perplexed me was that I didn't have a choice. Otherwise, I'd have been out of there faster than a seagull on a chip.

The pigeon had a choice. Its wings were in working order, yet it was just sitting there.

Tell me your secret, little pigeon. Why are you so content to sit still?

At that moment, I became a student of truth. I could no longer assume a starring role in my play, so I opted for being an observer, peeking from behind the open curtains. My world had come to a standstill, and I was alone for long stretches with nothing to preoccupy me but my thoughts. I found opportunities for mind wandering, reflection, and connecting the dots. Significant truths could be found by observing what was seemingly trivial and ordinary.

The pigeon was still because it was content. It had all it needed, safely perched up high with an endless supply of food and water below. It was in paradise and would not dare dream of leaving. I had all the same things the pigeon had. Lunch lovingly wrapped, waiting for me on the bedside table. Tom had tucked me into bed, where I was comfortable and warm. Yet instead of feeling like I was in paradise, I felt trapped between these four walls that resembled a prison. The bird knew the meaning of something I did not. It knew the meaning of "enough."

Admitting defeat, I moved onto exploring my defective senses. "Testing, testing, 1-2-3. La la la, mi mi mi." I sounded like a stranger to myself. I did not recognise my voice. I expected not to hear music, conversations, an aeroplane flying overhead, and other external sounds through my dead ear. I had not expected my own voice to be on that list. Turned out that being deaf meant not being able to hear internal sounds as well. When I spoke, it sounded like I was talking in an expansive cave, the sound echoey, distant, and distorted. This ghostly voice from another realm was so incredibly distracting that I felt barely present in conversations. I was unsure why I'd expected deafness to only apply to external sounds, but it caught me off guard. The list of strange sensations was endless. It was impractical for me to visit the doctor for every twitch, twang, and twinge I felt, so I simply had to ignore them or make up a plausible explanation to suppress my building hypochondria.

I compulsively swept away imaginary hair from my face throughout the day. My nerve damage made it feel as if there were stray hairs irritating my face or a spider crawling across my forehead. I began seeing floaters, little black dots suspended in my vision that floated about, dotting people's faces with moles they didn't have. Background images stopped updating in real-time and no longer bopped up and down with every step. I appeared to be gliding across the ground instead of walking. Random sharp pains deep in my ears, sometimes on the good side, jolted me out of whatever I was doing. The head pressure I felt was intense and unrelenting, as if a stern mistress had stacked several volumes of an encyclopedia on top of my head to promote perfect posture.

All these strange sensations made me acutely aware of my health, and it remained at the forefront of my mind. I kept thinking about what else was going to come for me without warning. What if my other ear suddenly stopped working too and my world became totally silent? How would my children communicate with me then? They were too young to read and write messages, and I would be cut off from them.

I would follow these paranoid thoughts down the rabbit hole until I filled myself with dread. Every tingle and feeling of numbness added to my hypochondria. From what I went through and what I learnt from others in the hyperbaric chamber, I knew all too well that what was in working order could break down in an instant. I had already used up my chance card and was operating with only one functional ear. There were still plenty of viruses waiting for me in the winds just outside my front door. I did not want to leave the house in case one caught me.

And what about all the other vital organs that I had only one of, such as the heart, liver, and brain? What if they suddenly failed too? My once safe world now felt fraught with unavoidable threats. I became hypervigilant to every danger cue. I started believing I was going to die. Every look and glance at my family was now through longing eyes, as I silently said goodbye, wishing for more time.

Every minute of the day, I felt as fatigued as if it was four in the morning as my brain worked hard to rewire itself. I spent my days in a daze, unable to focus or think. My brain was learning how to process an absence of the signals that used to come in from my left ear. The experts referred to this process as neuroplasticity. With no balance signals entering my brain from the left, any slight movement of my head was interpreted as rapid spinning. I had some control over being still during the day, consciously choosing to ignore the incessant nagging from my muscles begging me to move. During the night, however, my subconscious took over. Each time I changed position in my sleep, I got jolted back into consciousness, panicking, believing that I had just rolled off a building. Night after night, I was terrorised with the same. It was wearing me down.

I co-slept with our three-year-old daughter, Jade, due to her vulnerable health. She was less independent than Jet and had separation anxiety when I was not around. Since our little princess was born, we'd relegated poor Tom to the guest room.

One gung-ho night, I did a full turnover from back to belly. I awoke to violent vertigo, more dramatic than every other night. Whilst being spun at unimaginable speed in pitch darkness, I patted around for Jade. I wanted to scream for Tom to help but did not want to frighten Jade. Clinging onto her chubby legs, I waited for the tornado to pass. In slow motion, I sat up in bed and flicked on the bedside lamp. She was still deep asleep. I felt relieved that I'd somehow shielded her from what I was going through, at least this time. Amped up from the adrenaline yet simultaneously worn down in spirit, I sobbed uncontrollably and silently into my hands.

When there were no more tears to cry, my hands lowered into a prayer position. These palms had never before touched except to clap. I was a devout atheist. I have always been drawn to science and math, where unknowns could be proven. My need for concrete truth was the reason I elected to study engineering at university and had worked in the tech industry since graduating. I thrived in places where logic prevailed. However, in that moment, I was a desperate atheist and in dire need of a full night's rest. I broadcast my prayers out into the ether, hoping any merciful gods who were passing by would end my plight. "There are no atheists in the trenches" is a saying that's all too true at three thirty in the morning. I had no intention of falling asleep only to be terrorised again. I remained sitting in bed until sunrise.

Despite all this turmoil, each new day still brought with it new hope. The statistical line in the sand had been drawn at three months, after which all hope of recovery would be lost.

I still had one month left.

In that same week, Mormons knocked on my front door. I listened to them attentively and accepted their pamphlets. I even disclosed my mobile number. The last thing I needed was to offend a god. The Mormons must have put me on speed dial because their follow-up efforts to claim my soul were relentless.

"Why did you give them your number?" Tom questioned my out-of-character behaviour, clearly concerned for my sanity. However, this was not an isolated incident. Mum suggested I visit the temple for blessings to ease my suffering. To her surprise, I said, "Let's go!" In the last four decades, she had managed to drag me to the temple less than a handful of times, and that was to attend funerals or weddings. I lit incense sticks, got down on my knees, and ushered despairing words up to heaven with the smoke. Benevolent beings must live up there, I decided. I donated generously to the temple on the slim chance I could buy my way out of this predicament. I ate blessed foods, hoping for holiness to disperse through my broken body and work its miracles.

Every dawn was a disappointment. I woke up still deaf and dizzy. My spiritual quest had made no difference. If my Amazon Prime order could show up at my doorstep the very next day, surely I could expect my prayers delivered through divine logistics to be answered by now. The answers I was seeking could not be provided by any mortal being on earth. *Why me? What did I do to deserve this?* If I could just present a convincing case to the universe, my situation might just miraculously reverse itself.

I replayed my situation in my mind on a loop, covering different vantages. I critically examined myself from a moral deservedness standpoint. The worst I had done was break a few hearts before finding Tom. A classic goodie-two-shoes by every definition, I never smoked, never drank, and even steered clear of coffee in case it opened doors to stronger state-altering substances. As an adolescent, I was a straight-A student who beat Cinderella home every night so my parents could sleep soundly knowing their daughter was safely in her room. The moment I graduated, I earned my way entirely, paying taxes and sponsoring two children out of poverty and into education. I ate well, slept well, and led an active life. I did all the right things, made all the right choices, and ticked all the right boxes. Disability consequently seemed too severe a punishment for how I had carried myself to date. An unjust sentence ought to be reversed. If a reversal was not possible, maybe transference was.

Why me? turned into *Why not somebody else?* I formed my case, ready for a debate with the cosmos about why they should spare me. If I could just convince them I was the illogical choice, perhaps they would redirect my terrible fate elsewhere. I reasoned that I was a mum of two young children who needed me to be healthy and whole. My family relied on me as a co-breadwinner to keep a roof over our heads. This was a matter of survival. I was also our home's central processor, who organised and coordinated our activities. Lives would fall into disarray if I remained incapacitated.

I heard nothing back from heaven.

Chapter Five

Grasping at Straws

Hope is a good breakfast, but it is a poor dinner.
—*Francis Bacon, philosopher, statesman, and essayist*

Before long, my vulnerability decided it had had enough of binging on religion. God wasn't coming. It was up to me to make these horrible feelings go away. I shifted my focus to alternative medicines and supplements.

Through my constant motion sickness, I began reading, a sentence more each day than I could manage the previous day. I needed information on how to get better. I read mainstream journals for the latest in medical advancements—stem cell therapy, gene therapy, and other approaches to regenerate nerves. I researched alternative healing methods, including Ayurveda, energy healing and balancing chakras, grounding, meditation, reiki spiritual healing, and acupuncture. Inhaling marijuana and consuming Ayahuasca ventured too far out of my comfort zone, but I was willing to try everything else. I started with a variety of diets, from organic whole foods to smoothies loaded with antioxidants and superfoods. I even tried not eating, as intermittent fasting has been shown to place the body into repair mode. Salt went first on my elimination diet, followed by sugar, then caffeine. Besides losing a few kilograms, good food did little to repair my health. Arguably, our passion for cooking and gardening ensured we always ate well anyway.

When it came to supplements and vitamins, I bought and consumed the usual suspects, including vitamins C, D, and B complex, iron, magnesium, zinc, and calcium. A growing body of evidence indicates that gut health plays a vital role in our overall health, so I added probiotics and prebiotics to the regime. I even sourced magnesium L-threonate, the latest in magnesium discoveries, which can cross the blood-brain barrier to boost brain plasticity and encourage the formation of new brain cells. Given that all my problems were above the neck, it was worth a shot.

In my readings, I came across longevity studies by a renowned Harvard professor, Dr. David Sinclair, claiming that it was possible to reverse ageing—not simply tackle the visible signs of ageing, but truly stop time and even reverse it. It seemed inefficient to be addressing each symptom when I could eliminate them altogether by rewinding to a time when I was young and fit. Pricey NMN and resveratrol were added to my growing list of supplements. I must have spent thousands of dollars on vitamins and supplements, but I barely felt an energy boost, let alone any sense of being cured. My blood work prior to starting the supplements had come back within range, so perhaps I did not need them. Or perhaps the marketplace was stocked to the brim with snake oils peddled by charlatans, driven to do so by the capitalist system.

Besides popping handfuls of pills, my new morning routine consisted of standing under the shade of our apricot tree in the backyard, assuming Virabhadrasana, otherwise known as the warrior pose, and carrying out breathing exercises. According to Ayurvedic medicine, I was to inhale slowly, tracing my breath through my body and guiding it to the affected area. Don't ask me how. This breath, equivalent to being my life force, would move "stuck energy" along, which was preventing natural healing from occurring. I was then to exhale slowly, as if purging the body of impurities through the expelled air. The atmosphere was resonating at 432Hz, a healing frequency that I played during the exercises and, where practical, throughout the day. I supposed the routine was a kind of meditation. I would finish feeling calmer than before, with fewer visions of doom and gloom, if nothing else.

I could now move around slowly on my own and returned the walking frame to the hospital. I was a toddler learning how to walk, using the walls and furniture for support. On the way back to the house from the apricot tree, I often got distracted by our elaborate edible garden and meandered off course. People were frequently amazed at how we kept such a high-maintenance garden in check. I had a simple rule that every time we passed by the garden, be it to hang clothes or get to our cars, we had to pull a weed and plant a seed. But one day, as I leaned over to pull out an Oxalis and to plant a kale, my world turned upside down again. My face was the only organic matter that got planted in the ground that day.

"You have vertical benign paroxysmal positional vertigo," said the neurophysiotherapist during our weekly rehabilitation sessions. "It's common when people have experienced trauma in the inner ear. That's why you get a spinning sensation upon looking up or down." I immediately connected his explanation to the vertigo incident in the hyperbaric chamber when I'd dozed off and my head dropped.

The easiest way to describe the vestibular system is to imagine pretzel-like structures occupying a three-dimensional axis, perpendicular to one another. These structures are filled with sticky fluid and lined with motion-detecting nerves. When we tilt our heads, fluid moves over these nerves and they generate meaningful electrical signals to the brain, denoting our whereabouts in space. Right next to the vestibular system are otolith organs that have calcium crystals embedded in a gel-like substance resembling a sticky slice of gelatinous dessert. These crystals had become loose and found their way into my vestibular pretzel. Long after the fluids had settled from looking down, these crystals were still sinking to the bottom, brushing past nerves. Erroneous motion cues were then sent to my brain.

The neurophysiotherapist's job was to shepherd these loose crystals back to their otolith pens, hoping the gel gates would successfully contain them going forward. The only way to guide these calcium crystals through the pretzel maze was to place my head in a series of compromising and awkward positions for gravity to do its best work. Each turn of the pretzel triggered erroneous signals and vertigo ensued. It seemed awfully cruel that the only way to get rid of my frightening vertigo was to have me experience more frightening vertigo. I had to get sicker before I got better. Imagine telling a person with a broken leg to go walk it off. There would be a riot!

I endured those crystal ushering manoeuvres weekly for months as my anxious heart pounded away. My physical symptoms improved but never resolved. This came at the expense of deepening my trauma. Eventually, we were down to one allegedly stubborn horizontal canal that no fancy manoeuvres could cure. This meant I could not turn from left to right and vice versa whilst lying down, but I had been experiencing that all along.

While addressing my dizziness, I also visited a hearing centre to deal with my hearing issues.

"Sorry, you are not eligible for hearing aids," said the audiologist, examining my audiogram.

"I don't understand. I cannot hear anything. Why aren't I eligible?" I asked.

"Exactly. You have no useful hearing to work with. The aid needs something to amplify," she said.

Hearing aids are only available to ears that are hard of hearing, not to deaf ears. I was left with only two possible options. One was a CROS system, used to treat people with unilateral (one-sided) hearing loss. A microphone would be fitted on my broken side, which transmits signals to a receiver worn on my functional side. The privilege of picking up soft sounds on my deaf side, which would otherwise be blocked by the head shadow effect, would cost me six thousand dollars, not including periodic maintenance and replacement costs. Since my mobile phone frequently operated on one bar of battery, I could not imagine myself keeping these devices charged and in working order. It was a lot of kerfuffle and fiddly for a simple woman like me—make-up-free with a ponytail—who prefers squinting over wearing her glasses. I could hear well enough from anywhere in the room if the background noise was low. The gain was minimal for the price and effort.

My only other option was to have a cochlear implant. This involves invasive surgery to install a medical device that sends sounds directly to the brain. Should all go well, I would hear natural sounds from my working side and robotic sounds from my implanted side. This meant I would have Tom speaking in my right ear, and R2D2 in my left. For the cochlear implant to work, the auditory nerve to the brain must be intact. In the case of a damaged auditory nerve, the cochlear implant would be ineffective, necessitating a subsequent procedure to remove it. There was no way to tell if the implant would be successful until it was installed. It would set me back tens of thousands of dollars for the privilege of finding out.

A risk associated with this procedure is facial paralysis which would affect movement to half of my face and the ability to speak clearly and smile. There was also a risk of losing my taste, turning all foods into cardboard in my mouth. Finally, there was a risk that the vertigo would return.

After trading off risks versus rewards, I forwent the implant. The deal-breaker for me was the risk of returned vertigo. The thought of being bedridden again, unable to move, started my body rocking involuntarily. I couldn't go back there. And if the ultimate catastrophe were to occur, Jade was still too young to remember she once had a mother who loved her very much. Nothing was worth that.

Besides, I was medically compliant once with the experts. I took my excruciating steroid injections in the eardrums like a good girl. The injections never recovered my hearing. Instead, the pinprick left a weak chink in my eardrum armour. When I blew my nose, the chink tore and never healed. I now have a sizable perforation in my eardrum that forces me to sit out and watch while Jet and Jade splash around in a swimming pool with Tom, never to join them. I could opt to undergo surgery to repair my eardrum, but I drew the line. These medical interventions were like taking drugs to remedy the side effects of the original drug, and in doing so, trigger more side effects.

Parallel to modern Western medicine, I explored traditional Chinese medicine (TCM). The moment I stepped into the TCM doctor's practice, I was hit with nostalgic aromas of dried roots, leaves, and bark that reminded me of my late Chinese grandparents. They often had something similar brewing once upon a time. The doctor first soaked my feet in scalding herbal tea, then performed a process known as cupping. If you recall ever putting a drinking glass over your mouth as a child and sucking the air out of it, only to marvel as the glass remained stuck to your face when you took your hands away, cupping is a serious version of that. Instead of being left with a ridiculous ring around my mouth, which would fade by the end of the day, cupping left deep red and purple bruising all over my back. The vacuum created inside the cups drew blood to the surface of the skin and broke small capillaries. The idea was similar to the breathwork I had done under the apricot tree, which was to move qi, our vital life force, freely around the body. According to traditional Chinese medicine, blocked qi is the root cause of every imaginable ailment.

Qi, the doctor explained, moves along our central channel, which exists invisibly along the spine. This central channel is like a superhighway for energy to travel, with multiple turn-off exits, delivering essential qi to all parts of the body. If there is a blockage in the central channel, it puts the entire qi traffic system in jeopardy. To get energy flowing freely, the highway must be stimulated to clear it of debris.

The length of my spine was rubbed up and down vigorously until the skin was raw, priming my body for the next treatment—acupuncture. Acupuncture is yet another method of unblocking "stuck energy," but with precision, targeting specific locations. Cold sweat beaded at the thought of becoming a pincushion.

I lay down on an electrical pad that shot currents into my body, causing my muscles to spasm. Thread-like needles were pushed into me from head to toe to heal my ear. I was unsure what my feet had to do with my ear, and the doctor explained that traditional Chinese medicine believes in holistic healing. A weakness in one place may cause an illness in another. I had to be healed in totality.

The needles remained inserted for half an hour before I was told to flip over to begin on the other side. I rotated like a lamb roasting on a spit. Insertion of these several dozen needles was not painless, but it was tolerable, even for a wuss like me. My bravery was rewarded with a warm brew that looked and smelled suspiciously like what I had soaked my feet in earlier. *Anything that disgusting has to have medicinal properties*, I thought as I gulped it down. I left the wellness centre with several natural supplements that added to my already elaborate morning routine. I had six cupping and acupuncture treatments in total before I stopped, given the diminishing returns.

My situation had resulted in me searching hard for the silver lining without finding it. My mum had a Thai saying she would quote to me in times of despair. It translated to "Change misfortune into opportunity." I decided to put her teachings into practice. I rearranged the dinner table, placing my young children on my non-hearing side and Tom on my audible side. I had not had a more pleasant dinner in five years. Dual dialogues went on as usual with the children interrupting our conversation frequently, but this time, I could only really hear Tom's exchange. He had my undivided attention. I satisfied the children with my timely comments of "Ah huh" and "That's great," having no idea what they were talking about. This gave me an idea.

From then on, when my toddler had her tantrums, I carried and comforted her on my deaf side. Her gut-curdling screams seemed like they were happening miles away. As a result, she had a calmer and more compassionate mum by her side who settled her big emotions.

Extended sick leave allowed me to spend more time with my children. They stopped calling me by their nanny's name. Snortlepig stopped snorting altogether. Perhaps all a young child needed was his mother close by. I did not miss the rush-hour mayhem or picking the children up from care in the evening only to dash home, incessantly prompt them to swallow their dinner, hastily bathe them, and demand they fall asleep instantly. How was I ever satisfied with that? How did I ever feel that spending one hour with my children each day was enough? Since my illness, I had become more of a mother to them.

Then the day I dreaded came. From a medical standpoint, it marked the three-month milestone where all hope of further recovery would be lost. I had chased down every path to recovery, all to no avail. I had recovered no hearing and still could not take a stroll around the block unchaperoned.

I had been walking around the house with one earbud in, listening to "Pony" by Ginuwine on repeat for months because bass beats were the only sounds I could hear. Ginuwine was generous with the "burmfs" in "Pony". I was looking for any signs of improvements to my hearing, listening out for any noise that may have crept in between the "burmfs." Nothing. I gave up micro-monitoring my hearing because I could not bear to listen to another round of "Pony". It was self-inflicted psychological torture.

I joined a Facebook support group for those who have experienced sudden hearing loss, looking for any signs of hope that I could fan into manifestation. "Has anyone ever recovered from their total hearing loss after three months?" was the first post I wrote on their Facebook wall. A stream of supportive responses came back, each member expressing their sympathies and welcoming me into a group that no one would want to be part of. None reported recovering.

I had done enough mathematics in engineering to know that statistics only describe the general trend. There are always outliers that have beaten the odds, the long tail in distribution graphs. I could be one of them. There was always a first. In fact, I already had a track record of beating the odds.

"You are nearly thirty; shouldn't you be at home having babies instead of working?" I kept working. "You need to change the way you look. Kiddy rainbow ballerina flats do not lend themselves to a promotion." I was promoted. "You are five foot nothing, but when you meet with customers, stand like you are six feet tall." They nominated me as their preferred point of contact. I was the most unlikely candidate to be made a team lead, let alone an executive. A small Asian female with a polite, smiley demeanour had no place in a large, serious, British military organisation. The STEM field was male-dominated. I was the minority in every way, from race to gender to personality. Tom and I often joked that the only way I could be any more of a minority was to become a disabled lesbian. The irony was fierce, at least half of it.

There were one hundred thousand people across forty countries climbing this giant corporate pyramid. However, after two dedicated decades, I was a stone's throw away from the pinnacle, earmarked with the potential to keep going. The naysayers now were health statistics instead of men in suits. I just needed to focus and keep at it. I left my fate to hard work and time. Time, after all, allegedly healed all wounds.

Chapter Six

Choosing Life

Even the darkest night will end and the sun will rise.
—*Victor Hugo, writer, poet, and playwright*

It will be okay.
It's not going to be okay.
It will be okay.
It's not going to be okay.

I would pendulum between happily-ever-after optimism and an apocalyptic outlook. On good days, I felt like the heroine in my story. Any writer knows they could not kill the main character off this early in the piece. So it wasn't my time. There was more in store for me. This whole mess was just temporary, lasting long enough for me to learn some profound lessons. Once I had learned what I needed to, normality would return.

On bad days, I felt let down by sunrise. Opening my eyes and starting the day was drudgery, and I felt too dizzy to crawl out of bed and too deaf to care. I could only think of the brick wall wedged in my left ear and my bouncing vision. It was a different day, but the same woeful state. I felt resigned to my bleak future. If I showered that day, I was kicking goals. The in-between days were apathetic. For instance, I could take or leave ice cream, and I was usually a fiend for sweets.

I had now joined two Facebook support groups, one for vertigo and one for sudden hearing loss. There was no shortage of kind people reaching out privately, allowing me to vent. A little old lady was constantly checking up on me. Her picture was that of a classic granny: glasses resting at the end of her nose, grey head of hair tied in a neat bun, and surrounded by grandchildren. "How are you going, dear?" she would message. She introduced herself as having experienced sudden hearing loss several years ago. She told me that she converted her pain into purpose by reaching out and helping others. Healing other people had healed her.

For a couple of months, lengthy texting took place between me and this saint from Boston. She kept insisting

I share with her how I felt about my loss on the daily. As the weeks went by, my messages got shorter as I rehashed old feelings. There was a delicate balance between talking about feelings to get them off my chest and reinforcing the trauma through repetitive conversations.

I explained to the Boston Saint that I was no longer interested in talking about my traumatised feelings. It only stirred up the hornets' nest.

"How are you feeling today, dear?" the response read, and they kept coming. I stopped replying. Eventually, a message came that was loaded with red flags. It read, "All I want to do is to help people. I offer my time and my support to people like yourself and ask for nothing in return. It seems that my time is not worth your breath." I did not need another emotional burden and made a snap decision to block her. Several weeks later, I felt terrible, thinking I had been too harsh. I went to reinstate her and noticed her profile picture had changed. It was now of a pudgy, middle-aged man. She—or he—had catfished me. Clever, I thought, using a gender-neutral profile name. Working in information technology, I should have known better. And I did, but my vulnerability didn't.

People were breaking down in these forums over either their hearing loss or vertigo; I was experiencing both. But what we had in common was our inability to cope. Those who healed from their trauma or found ways to get on with life often left the group. What started as finding a kindred tribe that understood, fast became an echo chamber for misery. There were frequent posts on marriages breaking down from the pressure, and even a few "goodbye, cruel world" messages or notes to that effect.

In a conventional support group setting, had an attendee spent the session suggesting suicide, there would be a home follow-up from the counsellors. To use Facebook for any purpose without guardrails seemed irresponsible. The administrators were not trained counsellors, either. In the real world, this would have been equivalent to a hospital run by unqualified doctors who had watched a few episodes of *ER*. That would never be acceptable.

To their credit, the group administrators did warn they would report all suggestions of suicide to Facebook, but I doubted Facebook had a suicide intervention department. No Facebook negotiators were showing up on white horses to talk guns out of mouths. I could not tell with certainty how many suicide threats were followed through with. Perhaps the poster chose never to post again. Perhaps they could not post again, in which case, I hoped they'd found peace at last now that the screaming banshee in their head had been slayed. Mine was still shrieking.

I recall a post by a musician who had lost all hearing in one ear. He was in total despair and hung up his guitar for good. He could not bear to strum another note only to hear the disappointment. A woman in her early sixties who had been deaf since birth replied with her story. She had recently gotten a cochlear implant and was now hearing robotically out of one ear. Suddenly, she had access to conversations and sounds. She started taking piano lessons, elated by her new abilities. The musician was technically in a better-off position. He still had natural hearing in one ear, whereas she only had metallic hearing in hers. Yet their attitudes were as different as night and day. She had the wonderment of a child keen to engage with life, and he was depressed and withdrawn.

She addressed the Deaf community in her post, saying she'd been hesitant to get a cochlear implant because she was proud of Deaf culture and did not want to lose it. This culture was an expression of shared norms within the Deaf community, from rising above common challenges to the use of sign languages, and anything in between. She did not want to be ostricised by the only community she had ever known. Having now experienced both being deaf and partial hearing, she proclaimed that Deaf culture was not worth holding onto at the expense of hearing. The cochlear implant had improved her quality of life significantly.

Sure enough, the Deaf community began to lash out. It's a sad reality that health support forums are rife with comparisons and put-downs. In the healthy world, people compare successes. In the unhealthy world, people compare suffering. Sizing each other up never ends. It was this attitude that made me feel insecure about writing this memoir. I questioned whether my suffering was big enough, whether my misfortune was dramatic enough to warrant a book. Ridiculous, really. It did not matter in the end because just like the schoolyard days, no matter how big your daddy was, some kid always had a bigger daddy.

People have ended their lives for a lot more and a lot less than what I was going through. Not everyone is made equal, and we are shaped by our character and experiences. Being overwhelmed is a binary state. You are either coping, or you are not. Trauma happens when a tragedy surpasses a person's ability to cope. Trauma has no size. Rather, trauma is like light, capable of filling the entire room regardless of its wattage. No one's trauma is greater than that of another because the grief being felt is equal. The only difference is the story. Everyone's trauma journey is as individual as their fingerprints. Everyone has their cross to bear, and it is important to be kind.

My arrogance had me believing I got to my station in life through my own capabilities and hard work. The stories I heard through the Facebook groups made it clear now that the distance between having it all and living under a bridge was a short one. Many people shared their stories to receive support and lessen their pain. The trend was obvious. Losing their health had kicked off a domino effect. The suffering had robbed them of their cheery disposition and ability to work. For those who had a partner, dual-income households became one income. The family struggled under new financial pressures and living with a person they no longer knew, a person who was constantly unhappy. Marriages broke down. For the sufferer, one income often became no income. Going from having a family, health, and wealth to poverty, physical suffering, and being alone saw the most resilient people crumble and fall into an abyss, never to return.

I had been suffering for several months, and it was wearing me down. My ability to withstand hardship was eroded by this ordeal's unrelenting nature. It reminded me of the Twelve Apostles, a famous tourist attraction some five hundred kilometres away from my city. The attraction used to consist of twelve towering limestone columns that formed twenty million years ago. Driving on the road that wound parallel to the cliffs, it is possible to see these gigantic columns jutting out from the sea. When I was sixteen, my parents decided on a family road trip to witness this landmark. Upon arrival, I counted eleven apostles, not twelve. A column had collapsed a year earlier because of sea and wind erosion. What had withstood the test of time came tumbling down. Today, just eight apostles remain. Chip away at something long enough, and even the mighty and majestic will reach their limits. Like those fallen columns, I felt my tipping point was fast approaching.

School holidays commenced. My children became my shadows, following me in a line like ducklings. As a previously working mum, I had never been on my own with my children for this amount of time. Before my illness, Tom and I accrued the typical four weeks of annual leave while school holidays totalled a generous twelve weeks. We would take our leave together, which evened the odds: two adults versus two children. For the remaining leave discrepancy, Jet and Jade were off to family care. Now it made more sense for the children to be home with me since I wasn't working. One adult to two children was a shock to my system. With the skill sets and capabilities I had developed, it was easier to run a department than to look after two young children.

Jet and Jade screamed, laughed, shouted, and drummed up a racket, as children do. The louder the external noise, the more unbearable the internal noise became. Sirens wailed in my head without respite. One Saturday when Tom was home from work, he saw me run out of the house and into the garden. I stood under our apricot tree with my face in my hands. Tom followed me out. He clasped his hands around my wrists and lowered my arms. We locked eyes, mine welling with tears.

"How did I end up here?" I asked. "How did I go from the boardroom to cleaning food off the ground?" I looked up at him in despair, completely dissatisfied with my life.

"You are formidable, Nin, don't ever forget that," he began. "Make no mistake, you are a warrior in the garden."

I knew exactly what he meant because I had heard this concept before, and it was even more fitting that I was standing in our garden. A disciple of Bruce Lee, who was training in kung fu, asked the master, "Why do you ask us to train every day but teach us not to fight?" The master replied, "It is better to be a warrior in a garden than a gardener at war." The meaning of the story is that one should be prepared for hardship even during peaceful times because adversity is inevitable.

To apply it to my context, Tom meant that I had suddenly found myself in a garden. I was no longer sparring with worthy opponents in an arena, or in my case, no longer working towards worthwhile goals with colleagues at the office. He encouraged me to train during this downtime in the garden, that I should continue to read, learn, and grow while I was not working. I had been an avid reader who no longer picked up a book. I was a curious learner who no longer asked questions. Not working did not mean I had to become a gardener, slipping into the world of children and mind-numbing household chores. I could remain a warrior. I just needed to train again.

When I was living with Mum and Dad in my early twenties, we had neighbours who were in their nineties to the left, right, and directly opposite us. They had no need to move to a retirement village because our street already resembled one. They would sit on their porches soaking up the first sunlight, putter around in their gardens, and go about their days, albeit slowly. *How are they so calm?* I'd thought to myself. They knew they had a death sentence coming any moment now. I expected them to be nervous wrecks, popping anti-depressants like Tic Tacs. I would not be able to function if I was told with certainty that any day soon could be my last. I wouldn't be able to sleep just in case I transitioned to the Pearly Gates that night. I had just taken out a loan for a shiny new sports car, and I hadn't even met my future spouse yet. The idea of my demise was unfathomable. My elderly neighbours, however, appeared unphased by their impending doom.

I used to think old people were just ready to go, having done everything and seen everything, so there was nothing left to hang around for. After experiencing my health trauma, I realised this was not the case. Wanting to go or stay is a delicate balance between how much you have to live for versus how difficult it is to live. Based on where the scales landed determined whether you threw yourself at life or started knotting the noose. Where I was on my journey, pain outweighed pleasure. Every day was arduous to see through to the end. Even walking felt like it was done through treacle. Without balance and proper hearing, nothing was easy. I was no longer eager to be here.

I imagined my neighbours had felt similarly, and most certainly had more than me to deal with—knobbly knees, rickety hips, diminishing senses, comorbidities, chronic fatigue, and all-over aches and pains, both emotional and physical. They would have had to say goodbye to family and friends along the way. Their world was no longer Eden. I suspected that death wasn't scary because they had already lost the will to live. I sure couldn't live the rest of my life like this. Things had to get better, or they had to end.

After several weeks of contemplating both options, I made my decision on one unsuspecting night. Jade had fallen asleep before me, as she always did. She was lying on her side facing me. Still unable to move much, I turned over slightly and side-eyed her. In the soft glow of my phone light, I could see her round, peaceful face, completely unbothered by the world. I reached out to hold her hand. The mind's ability to envision the future before it happens is a "try before you buy" arrangement we all have access to. I imagined what it would feel like if I closed my eyes permanently. I took in the details of Jade's face, every curve, every line, and closed my eyes. In less than a minute, I wanted to open them again just to see her. I overruled my instincts and kept them closed. Before long, it felt like my head was being held underwater. To see Jade would be to draw the breath I needed. She alone was a powerful enough reason to live. I had too much to live for; I wasn't going anywhere!

The next morning, I shared with Tom my epiphany that I'd had deep in the darkness of night. "You better get busy living then," he replied. He turned back to follow up with, "You could be a vegetable in hospital, and if we got to hug you every week, it would be better for all of us than losing you. Just letting you know in case you want to consider our opinions next time."

My strategy was set. I chose to live. I chose to be a warrior in the garden. It was time to "burn the boats," a phrase often used in management for extreme commitment to plan A because there was no plan B. Great leaders in the past, including Alexander the Great, have deployed the burning of the boats as a war tactic to motivate their troops and make it clear there was no possibility of retreat, that victory was the only acceptable outcome.

I had days where I thought I was going to emerge victorious and days where I thought I would never make it. I was confused about whether I was getting better or getting worse, whether I was dealing with it or not. Healing from trauma was not a linear journey. I had been healing since I left the hospital after my acute episode. I had also been hurting as the hope of recovery dwindled. Healing and hurting were two independent processes that ran parallel to one another, locked together in an arm wrestle. It could go either way on any given day. My grief graph was like that of the stock exchange, up and down, but ultimately, it began trending up the moment I chose life. I was a smidgeon less sad that day than I was the day before, though not enough to notice. However, the law of small gains states that consistent incremental improvements will inevitably lead to monumental results.

Chapter Seven

Invisible Change

It is very unfair to judge anybody's conduct, without an intimate knowledge of their situation.
—*Jane Austen, novelist*

I had been keeping to myself a lot after what happened, but the arrival of spring weather encouraged me to put on my walking shoes and take a stroll at the local reserve. I knew it would be good for me. Everything that could go wrong ran through my mind, but I mustered enough courage to follow through with the plan. The weather was mild, but the sun still felt warm on my skin. It was the tranquillity I needed to straighten out my jumbled thoughts.

"Well done," I said to myself. "You got out of the house."

Before long, my thoughts were interrupted. DING DING! DING DING! I frantically looked around for the source of urgency when it zoomed past me. The bicyclist leaned over and yelled, "Get out of the way, you fucking idiot!" Startled, I hopped off the trail, fighting back frightened tears. Having one audible ear meant I had lost sound direction and was not aware of him approaching from behind. He did his part by ringing the bell. I did not do mine by moving out of his way. When his reasonable expectation was not met, I was judged, in his words, as a "fucking idiot."

Had I been hobbling on crutches with one leg in a cast, I would like to think he would have accommodated me by simply riding off the track briefly and leaving it at that. Or perhaps if everyone was like me and could only hear out of one ear, the protocol for cyclists would be to ring their bell and shout out their location, such as, "Right behind you," and all would be well. Instead, I was exposed as a fraud, trying to fit in with a healthy and able society. I now lived in a world that was no longer made for me; it was made for the able. I no longer felt normal here.

Invisible disabilities and illnesses, including mental health issues, are prevalent in our communities. Those of us affected live amongst the able, shopping where they shop, dining where they dine, and working where they work. It is difficult for us to advocate for our needs in a system that relies upon tangible proof. Doctors hold back prescriptions and insurers hold back their approval because even trained professionals are sceptical of invisible conditions. When we are exposed as frauds trying to fit in, we attempt to explain our condition to people. They will be disbelieving, though, as if everything is occurring in our messed-up minds and it's nothing an attitude adjustment couldn't fix. Eventually, we grow so tired of explaining ourselves and trying to fit in that we withdraw from society. To live isolated and alone is often the fate of people with an invisible illness or disability.

I thought back to earlier days when I still had my walking frame at the supermarkets, when my disability was visible. I did not fit in with people's expectations then either. They stared, possibly reconciling in their minds why a relatively young woman with no wounds or even a limp would depend on a walking frame.

It appeared I had two choices: to visibly show my struggles and be met with gawking sympathy, or to conceal them and be met with cruel ignorance. I have always hated being in the limelight, even on my birthday. Suffering in silence was more my style, so invisible disability it was. The cyclist's insult was not going to take away my small win of getting myself out of the house. I needed to keep pushing back against the boundaries that had been closing in.

My next challenge was to drive again. Tom had been the only parental pillar precariously holding up our family since I became sick, driving us around everywhere. I was desperate to feel useful again and even more so to ease his burdens. My knuckles turned white as both hands tightly gripped the steering wheel. I peered out onto the main road. Roads I had negotiated with ease for decades were now the Wild West and looked like total mayhem. I took a deep breath to dispel my nerves, and for the first time in several months, joined the stream of cars on their commute. My compact SUV had transformed itself into a hovercraft. At least, that was how it appeared to drive—suspended off the road, bobbling up and down, navigating a three-dimensional space.

In hindsight, I was a danger to myself and others on the road. Without fluid movement of my head or the ability to determine sound direction, I was driving with an impairment. There were laws to prevent drink driving, but there were no laws to prevent driving while as dizzy as a drunk. Or if there were such laws, no one pointed them out to me. The hospital simply told me to return home and get on with life. Besides, at that moment, I didn't care. I was no longer held prisoner at my address. The sense of freedom that came from being behind the wheel was the liberating rain to my stranded desert.

I justified my reckless behaviour since I wasn't going far. I was just doing a school pick-up a few minutes' drive from where we lived. I had not done one of these for months. Soon after I arrived, the classroom door burst open on the bell. When Jet saw me, his starry eyes lit up. With arms stretched wide, he charged towards me, screaming, "Mummy!" It was the mood booster I needed.

Life could only be held back for so long before its natural inclination to move forward overpowered its anchors. When you were sick for a week, loving family and friends could be expected to step in and fill the gaps. When you were chronically ill, there came a point where life moved on, dragging you behind it whether you were ready or not. School pick-ups were straightforward enough and therefore were the ideal responsibility to resume first. I dreaded the bigger challenges, such as caring for Jade around the clock during an asthma attack, and it was only a matter of time before one happened. Would I be able to handle it?

That day came when I watched from the kitchen window as my energetic daughter played outside with her brother. Anyone would be hard-pressed to tell that she had any underlying conditions at all. She could run all day through flower fields in spring and never be short of breath. She smashed through her developmental milestones. Her paediatrician requested an IQ test. The results revealed what he had suspected—she was in the high genius range. By every marker, she was a superhuman child, yet the hospital classified her as a vulnerable person. To me, she was not vulnerable. Rather, she had her one kryptonite—the common cold.

Jade came inside after playing with her brother. She sneezed. Tom and I froze. Dread washed over us. We knew what would come next. To most people, catching a cold was a normal part of life, a slight inconvenience to be dealt with now and again. I too thought as such until Jade came along. She contracted her first respiratory virus at four months old, which landed her in the emergency department. As a naturally small infant, it was particularly concerning for doctors when she stopped eating and drinking. Not long after arriving at the hospital, she closed her eyes. I'd watched them remain closed for three long days while I circled her cot. My heart shrivelled at the pitiful sight of her tiny frame connected to cables and tubes. Jade was diagnosed with virus-induced asthma. That meant she struggled to breathe each time she contracted a run-of-the-mill respiratory virus.

It was no different this time. Her hospital bag was always packed and ready to go. I watched over her tirelessly throughout that night, monitoring her chest rising and falling, evaluating the sound of her breathing. It was always hard to decide when to start the mad dash to the hospital. If I called it too soon, they would send us back home, having wasted precious resources that could have been used to save another life. If I called it too late, we would lose our daughter. At two in the morning, I made the executive decision to load up the car. I had to be the one who accompanied Jade to the hospital, as I had been doing so for the last three years. It was me who knew the routine and what to do should she regress along the way.

Tom paced slowly towards the car as I reversed carefully out of the driveway with Jade seated in the back. I could barely drive a few blocks during the day. How was I going to drive to the central business district under the cloak of night? To a normal person, it would be a non-event. To me, it was stunt driving. I might as well have been leaping over ten cars that were lit on fire. My face must have looked full of terror. I began to hyperventilate. I locked eyes with Tom. Although the drizzly windshield camouflaged my tears, he knew. He always knew. And so the conservative man I married, who kept his T-shirt on even at the beach, swiftly took it off and swung it around over his head in the freezing night rain. I smiled at the unexpected *Magic Mike* moment. Uncontainable laughter ensued, breaking my funk.

I whispered, "Mummy and Daddy got you, little Jade. All you've got to do is keep breathing."

Upon arriving at the hospital, they ushered us in immediately. The rescue window is small; people cannot survive for long without air. Jade needed saving with drugs that could only be administered by medical professionals.

I sat slumped in a nearby chair as medics fussed over her. A kind nurse approached me and said, "Children are anxiety-inducing, aren't they? Don't worry; she will be okay. We see lots of kids like her every day." Her voice was the warm hug I needed. In her fairy godmother-like presence, I wanted to tell her everything: That I was constantly on the verge of tears. That I could not cope. I wanted to share what had happened to me. That I felt unwell, and I too ought to be a patient in this hospital. I wanted to confess that I was drowning. That I had resumed my role as a parent but was no longer made from the same stuff. That I was weak and crumbling inside.

"Thank you," I replied instead.

Jade was fast asleep in my arms by the time we were admitted to our ward. As I watched her sleep, I thought about our intertwining fate, mother and daughter. Here I was struggling in the aftermath of a cold, lying beside my child who was fighting to live because of the same. Unlike Jade, my childhood had been blessed with exemplary health. I was not classed as vulnerable or immune-compromised. I did not even have allergies. I barely missed a day of school or work for four decades. I felt invincible, which made it even more unimaginable that a common cold would change my life forever. Perhaps I was just unlucky. Or perhaps catching a cold was a game of Russian roulette, where each spin brought the players closer to the unthinkable.

Having been healthy for most of my life, I had paid little attention to the vulnerabilities of others until Jade was born. Her condition made me aware that there were many other people like her. On her first admission to the hospital with breathing troubles, I was told that at least one in ten Australians had asthma. In the days before Covid-19, Jade, and labyrinthitis, catching a cold did not change my routine. I still went to work, caught public transport, and attended parties. I was oblivious to the detrimental impact I could have had on vulnerable people until I saw Jade struggle with a common cold. People on ventilators fighting for their lives had caught their respiratory virus from somebody. Jade and I caught our colds from somebody. I thought about how many people I could have maimed or even killed without knowing just by being out and about with a cold. I used to be able to sleep soundly at night without giving it a second thought because tracing fingerprints on weapons was easier than tracing signatureless viruses in the air.

The soft glow of early morning light seeped into the room. I felt relieved that I could still care for Jade in my compromised state. I had been concerned that I would not hear her faint wheezing, preventing me from attending to her needs. Visions of her slipping into unconscious oblivion from oxygen deprivation weighed on my mind. Yet, somehow, we made it through the night. Her cries, rather than her difficult breathing, alerted me to her discomfort. I used to administer her puffer when her wheezing arose, allowing her to continue sleeping. Now she had to wake and cry to prompt my attendance. Though not ideal, it wasn't game over.

After breakfast, a respiratory specialist visited Jade. She had a background in immunology and cautioned us to stay away from large crowds when possible. It was not in Jade's best interest to catch a cold, given the predictable complications that followed. I questioned whether avoiding viruses would be detrimental to the healthy development of her immune system. Like many others, I was led to believe that being exposed to viruses was good for us. I believed the exposure would result in the formation of immune memory, where the body learns to recognise viruses it has encountered before and better defend itself against them.

She smiled and said, "You can catch the same cold three weeks later and end up back here. We see that often. Keep her away from sick people and crowds. She may grow out of this. Give her some time."

In response to our cautious attitudes, people often told us, "Catching a cold is good for kids' immune systems," sometimes even advocating for childcare centres as the means of acquiring the goods. Knowing what we knew now through our lived experiences and many rounds of consultations with respiratory and immunology specialists, saying a cold was good for the immune system was as ludicrous to me as saying that bullying was good for character building. There were better ways to achieve the same results without the risks of downtime and health complications. These ways included healthy foods, fresh air, exercise, and plenty of sleep, to name a few. I thought about how our hunter/gatherer ancestors lived sparsely in small tribes, not congregating by the millions in dense cities and being bombarded with viruses from all angles. We still have their biology today. Surely, our immune systems were not designed to handle this many viruses.

After Jade was born, our social circle split into two: those who understood and respected our boundaries when it came to Jade getting sick, and those who did not. We saw the second group a lot less. There were no harsh feelings on our side. Our road simply forked from theirs, fated by our circumstances, and we chose to put protecting Jade first. Surprisingly, the Covid pandemic was the best thing to have happened to our family. It turned the perception of cautious people who believed in preventative measures—like us—into caring and considerate people, which became the norm out of necessity. In turn, those who were relaxed and used to taking their snotty selves out everywhere had to consider their decisions more carefully, lest they be thought of as inconsiderate. For once, the script was flipped in our favour. We were no longer the over-cautious lunatics.

The hospital discharged Jade, but her breathing was still wet, evidenced by the wheezing and crackling. She was, however, out of imminent danger. No longer working, I felt thankful I could be home taking care of her, instead of rushing her back to childcare.

That same week, we were supposed to take a road trip. We had planned it with our extended family long before all this chaos unfolded. It was a special event that marked a significant milestone for one of our family members. We wanted to be there to show our support. However, the thought of being in a forest retreat, hours away from the nearest hospital with no ambulance access, was concerning. My family had become dependent on hospitals, and now we would have to leave our security blanket behind with the city.

Tom and I had taken our children to Silverton several times before, just the four of us. It was a picturesque area south of the city, with rolling hills along the way. Lush green forests surrounded the area to one side and pristine seas on the other. It was an ideal place for hiking, fishing, and reconnecting with nature. At the right season, when the weather was warm, every step through the grassy meadows sent a kaleidoscope of monarch butterflies up in every direction. Our children would scream with delight as they chased the monarchs, only to have more fluttering wings fill the air with every step. To be there was to be in a dream.

The long drive this time was vastly different from how I remembered it. The journey was the same—it was me who had changed. Verdant green sceneries were now muted in colour, as were the once bright blue skies. The sprawling countryside that had felt peaceful now seemed lonely and depressing. The joyful music playing in the car was an awkward party where everyone was dancing while I sat out with my two left feet. My tinnitus roared to match the volume of the stereo.

Eventually, we arrived at our destination. The moment I stepped out of the car, I was hit with terrible disequilibrium. I was starting to hold my own walking on flat surfaces in the city, but sloping hills and uneven soil proved to be a challenge.

Everyone was keen to set off hiking, as the views were promised to be spectacular. Jade could not run three steps without gasping for air, having not yet recovered from her acute asthma attack. I could not trust my feet to take me anywhere, let alone down an unfenced, windy mountain with uneven terrain. Unaccustomed to being the party poopers, we agreed to go along. Jet shot off like a bloodhound on a scent. Tom instinctively ran after him. If anyone were to jump off the cliff just to see what would happen, it would be our rambunctious five-year-old son. His combination of intelligence, restlessness, and bravery made Jet a classic case of curiosity killed the cat waiting to happen.

In his five short years, his shenanigans have given us plenty of material to roast him with when he turns eighteen. He has ripped the legs off a redback spider, the most venomous spider in Australia, a country notorious for animals that can kill you. The redback bit him right back, to be fair, sending him screaming and tearing his hair out to the emergency department. The neurotoxins had activated every pain receptor in his body. Anti-venom had to be administered. But wait, there's more. He once leapt to begin his gymnastic, single-bar routine. The only problem was that the bar belonged to his sister's pram, which was locked into position. The force of his swing pivoted the pram, sending three-month-old Jade catapulting through the air, landing like a starfish on our hardwood floor. Another time, he set a leather couch on fire at an Airbnb, resulting in a lifetime ban for us. Oh, and he has tangled himself in a barbwire fence. We had to unpick his skin to set him free. He has toppled a bench press onto himself, only to be saved from death by his skinny frame that rested just below the bar bearing the weights. Thank goodness he was a fussy eater. He also did a run-up onto a moving escalator, and upon landing, busted his knee open on a metal step. He stacked chairs to bypass our pool fencing security, leading Jade, who did not have the ability to swim, to fall in. That was why the scruff of his neck needed to be within Tom's reach at all times on this hike.

Jade and I hiked at a less suicidal rate than the boys, but it still felt like I was walking a tightrope. With my impaired vestibular system, I was certain I could be blown off this mountain by a breeze. We did not venture far before Jade's asthma played up again. My heart sank to see her work so hard at breathing. We were in the middle of nowhere. No rescues were coming if she stopped breathing now. I picked her up to deter her from huffing and puffing. I was now walking a tightrope with a fifteen-kilogram sack of potatoes. We quickly fell behind the rest of the group. The hikers in front grew smaller and smaller until we could no longer see them. Clouds moved in and drizzled rain, muddying the surface. My shoes no longer guaranteed traction, and I had no arms available to cushion any potential falls. Enough was enough. I was reluctant to take on any more risks and sat us down on a stool-shaped rock.

"Mummy, get up and keep going. I don't want to be last," Jade pleaded, whipping her horse with her words.

"I'm sorry, Jade. Mummy just can't."

I sang songs, scratched her back, and played clapping games with her to lift her spirits. There was no mobile reception in the outback, so I could not call Tom. We waited until Tom had caught Jet and doubled back for us. After sizing up the hike, he knew neither of us was in a condition to get very far. Tom saw his wife and daughter sitting out, defeated. Jade was still solemn from missing out on the fun adventure, and I was gutted by the scorn on her face because I could not carry her to the end. Jet threw a tantrum, adding to my guilt. He wanted to know what was waiting at the finishing line.

"We don't need to hike! I know a place where there are plenty of kangaroos," suggested Tom. With those words, Jade sprang back to life and Jet calmed right down.

We spent the afternoon together, just the four of us, exploring flat lands and lush green meadows just like when we came here in the past. True to his words, we spotted a mob of kangaroos. There were around a dozen does with joeys peeping out of their pouches. Bucks stood nearby, acting as bodyguards, so we kept our distance. They were bigger than Tom, and he stood six feet tall with broad shoulders. The last thing our family needed was another reason to go to the hospital, this time with the headlines that read "Man vs Kangaroo."

Tom turned to the children and boasted, "You know I could take them all on, but we need to be respectful of animals."

That night, we hosted dinner for our extended family at our retreat. As I listened to their tall tales of victory from the hike, I could not help but wonder if we were completely unseen. If brothers, sisters, mothers, and fathers could not see our struggles from up close, how could we expect the rest of the world to? To be fair, we appeared normal, had colour on our cheeks, and even put on a delicious meal. Perhaps if we had a tell like

Jade's oxygen tubes or my walking frame, they might have selected an alternative activity to the hike.

From that day, I stopped spending energy blending in with the healthy and able society, knowing in my heart that I was a fraud. Now and then, I'd be exposed for my dishonesty, such as by the cyclist, and now by our family. I did not want to anchor anyone back from doing what they wanted, but nor did I want to feel pressured to do what we could not. We removed ourselves to live life at our own pace. We chose to be a happy family in a field of kangaroos.

Chapter Eight

Lost Hope and Dashed Dreams

Happiness, not in another place but this place, not for another hour but this hour.
—*Walt Whitman, poet*

I caught Jade's cold and was struck with fear that the virus would go wandering off again. I could not shake the cold for several weeks and was having trouble breathing. The doctor confirmed there was crackling and wheezing in my lungs. I was not an asthmatic, so drowning from the inside was a new sensation to me. The doctor was concerned that my prolonged cold would lead to pneumonia and prescribed a broad-spectrum antibiotic. When I finished the course and was no better, she prescribed a targeted antibiotic and asked me to return in three days. Again, I was no better. She then put me on yet another antibiotic. I was now taking both simultaneously. The medication was wreaking havoc on my body, and I still felt like I was swallowing a cactus. I decided not to go back for my fourth dose of antibiotics. I was prepared to go straight to the emergency department if my condition escalated to pneumonia. Between my and Jade's problematic health, I could drive there blindfolded by now. A lingering cold was the least of my problems when compared to the grief I was going through.

It had been four months since the onset of labyrinthitis. What I had lost was still a constant in the forefront of my mind. It consumed me. Thoughts of hearing loss and dizziness interrupted my conversations and activities more than a needy toddler. Not a minute passed without me thinking about my deafness. I'd be cooking ... *deaf*. Eating ... *deaf*. Showering ... *deaf*. Driving ... *deaf*. Tidying ... *deaf*. I could not escape the awareness. The absence of sound was the opposite of silence. The tinnitus was unbearable.

Unlike my subtle obsession with not hearing, my obsession with balance was evident and visible. Every few minutes, I would place my head in a provocative position just to experience the whoosh. I did this more often than a nervous wreck bit their nails. I'd look up at different angles, hoping for a pleasant surprise, that the disequilibrium would have gone away. It never did. It whooshed every time. We were out in public when Tom pointed out discreetly, "You're looking strange."

Unilateral hearing came with many drawbacks. Loss of sound direction and tinnitus were the obvious two. What became apparent later was that I could no longer focus on individual sounds. Similarly to how eyes can focus on an object and blur out the peripherals, the ears can do the same regarding sound. In noisy restaurants where forks and spoons clank incessantly, a normal hearing person can pull out the conversation they are having, distinguishing it from the background noise. I couldn't. I had lost the ability to focus on sounds in busy environments. Restaurants being the social scene of choice for much of society, I may as well have been totally deaf in them. This narrowed down my options for meeting people to build meaningful relationships to my house or theirs. The introvert in me would have been fine with this, but the dedicated foodie in me was not. Escargot braised in parsley butter, crab linguine with a dash of cream and chilli, crusty garlic naans baked in traditional tandoori ovens, and lamb tagine with preserved lemon in every bite—all were no longer easily accessible to me. As a result, I dreamt of food often.

Excessive background noise in supermarkets was merciless. On one occasion, I wheeled my trolley full of groceries to the checkout and the lady behind the counter said something inaudible. I could not lip-read, but I knew instinctively that she was asking if I needed bags since they had to ask that. I said, "Yes, please." After putting the groceries through, she moved her lips again. I produced my Visa card to pay. Our transaction finished with her saying something else. I replied, "Thank you. You have a nice day too." My responses must have been spot on, judging from the smooth transaction and her unphased reaction. I left the shops feeling uninspired, knowing that anyone could have had this successful exchange on either side of soundproof glass. Routines and systems seemed to have killed off meaningful human connections in the name of efficiency. If I could hear conversations in supermarkets again, I would shake things up. I'd buy her a drink and ask her about her day.

The wetness in my lungs dried up, replaced by a nasty cough that tore up my chest muscles. It hurt to even breathe. I had to take in air like I would sip water—in small puffs. I had been sick for months with a virus or viruses that made themselves at home in my body, yet no one else in the family had caught it off me. We lived and ate together daily, not to mention the smooches. Only my immune system was compromised to that extent. My body was now benefiting from a slower, stress-free pace and an elaborate vitamin-supplement regime. I was on extended sick leave and had plenty of leisure time for walks in the sun and cooking wholesome meals. My body should have been repairing itself, not breaking down.

Spring weather enticed me out for many walks around the block with the children. That was the extent of my bravery in venturing out. I preferred to be a close kilometre or two from home and was now living life through the "just in case ..." lens. One walk stood out more than the others. It was a calm walk full of cute conversations.

"Mummy, what is the most powerful thing on Earth?" Jet asked. All things mighty fascinated him.

I thought for a moment and said, "Time. Time is the most powerful thing on Earth."

He tried to wrap his brain around my answer and poked at my theory. Jet could take nothing at face value. He needed to get to the bottom of everything. His insatiable curiosity drove Tom and me up the wall.

"What about the strongest man in the world?" Jet asked.

To which I replied, "In eighty years, he won't be here. He will grow old and die."

Jet continued to brainstorm. "What about an erupting volcano then?" he asked, looking up at me with inquisitive eyes.

"It would eventually run out of steam. In a few months, the volcano would hardly be anything more than an inert mountain. Time is still the most powerful, son."

There was a long pause as we kept walking. Jet turned to me and asked his most poignant question. "What about deafness, Mum? Time has not made that go away."

I choked, searching for an answer that never came.

We continued our walk along the pedestrian path. I had my working ear facing the road to listen out for traffic. I felt safer that way. My broken side faced the houses. As we turned the corner, we were ambushed by thunderous, rapid barking. My instincts took over, telling me to flee from the danger. In a flash, I grabbed both children and pushed them straight into the snout of an aggressive canine protruding from a barred fence. My kids screamed as they lunged to get away. The dog had been barking on my left side, the side that could no longer hear. Given I could only receive sound from my right, I thought the dog was to our right. I had misjudged the dog's whereabouts in a fight-or-flight instant and delivered my children into the jaws of the beast.

"I'm so sorry, kids," I exclaimed. "I thought the dog was on the other side."

They looked at me like I had gone mad. I surveyed them from top to bottom for any scratches or bites. The near miss rattled me to the core. A mother's primary job, above education or providing comfort, was to keep her children safe. I had failed. I would never have forgiven myself had they been bitten. My confidence in being a mum plummeted at the realisation that I could no longer protect my children.

Not only was I unable to protect my children physically, but I could not protect them psychologically. It had come to my attention that my children were worried about me and were expressing it in different ways. Jet was contemplating whether deafness was more powerful than time. Little Jade started leaning into my dysfunctional ear nightly at tuck-ins. I knew from the warmth of her breath pitter-pattering on my skin that she was whispering a message to me.

"You know I can't hear from that ear. You must speak to the side with no mole," I explained one night, pointing to the predominant beauty spot on the left side of my face that served as a marker for my broken ear.

"I know, Mummy," she replied. "I wanted to speak to your deaf ear." Confused, I questioned why. She replied, "I asked it to get better because I don't want my mummy to be deaf anymore."

A current shot through my chest. Innocent growing brains were supposed to be filled with wonder, not be preoccupied with my adult issues and misery.

"Jade, what can I not do with you that I could do with you before? What does it matter that I'm deaf? I don't care. Why should you?" I inquired, playing it down. I was gauging how I might have slipped in my duties as a mum. Nothing should have changed for her. We still ate ice cream together, walked to the playground together; I still read to her and drank many cups of her imaginary tea.

"Deaf makes you so sad, Mummy. I don't want you to be sad anymore," Jade said with downcast eyes.

Jet and Jade's preoccupation with my troubles prompted me to better hide what I was going through. I did not want it to affect them. The roles were reversed, and it felt wrong. I was supposed to worry about my children, not the other way around. I started smiling again, wide and often, hoping to fool a three- and a five-year-old with my plastic grin. It worked better than expected. I fooled not just them but everyone. I was still full of sorrow, but outwardly, I now looked like society expected me to, like I was healing and moving on.

It was difficult to be truly happy when my dreams had been shattered and the lights dimmed on my once bright future. Three weeks before I ended up in the hospital, Tom and I were standing on top of a misty hill, hand in hand, admiring twenty acres of charming country estate.

"Just imagine having our breakfast right here, darling," I said, giddy with joy, seeing in my mind's eye a steaming cup of tea against the hazy backdrop.

"I'm going to stock that dam full of redfins. Jet and I will catch us dinner," Tom said with a grin, staring out into the distance, lost in his vision.

On the small suburban block that we still called home, we had ripped up our lawn and replaced it with rows upon rows of vegetables. Each morning, the children would collect eggs from our faithful hens and pick their snacks for the day—tomatoes, cucumbers, and sugar snap peas were their favourites. We wanted to expand our lifestyle, but there was no room left. A hobby farm seemed the natural progression of our passion. We put forward our best offer to the real estate agent and kept our fingers crossed.

Wild emus stormed our property-to-be as we made our way back to the car from the open inspection. They towered over Tom in height. The quintessential Australian thing to do when challenged by emus was to make a beak with our hands and lift our arms high above our heads. We pretended we were bigger emus, intimidating them right back. Our short stacks had no chance at pretending to be the alpha bird and clung onto each of Tom's legs in fear, bolstering his presence. Success. We parted the Red Sea of emus and made our way through. We laughed till our bellies hardened at our soon-to-be crazy country life.

"Fixing that fence is going to be my first job. We can't have emus coming in and attacking the kids," Tom had said as he continued to plan.

Those beautiful daydreams became pipedreams overnight. We called the real estate agent and withdrew our offer the week I was in hospital. He was sympathetic to our situation and let us off the hook. I could barely run a humble household, let alone an acreage. Still, we were outgrowing our tiny home that I had bought as a single graduate. I had always thought this would be a transitional abode, and when I met my soulmate, I believed we would get married and buy our forever home together. It did not happen that way. We got too comfortable. Now married with two kids in tow, we had marginally more space than battery hens. We still needed a solution for growth but were now absent of direction with the tree change taken off the table. Worse, should I not be able to return to work, we were no longer certain of our financial means to expand. Plans that had been meticulously laid out step by step were uprooted. Our future was now a blank screen marked with a single blinking cursor. Tom and I could not agree on a first word for our new story. The thought of a suburban life with perhaps an extra bedroom or two was a piercing arrow to his heart. What happened to me did not just end my dreams, it ended his as well.

I continued to live out groundhog days with no direction of expansion or growth. I passed my days by strolling the streets close to home. We used to be a travelling family that loved to explore, learn, and experience cultural novelty. I would feel jittery if I did not jet off several times a year. I still felt those confinement jitters, but there was nothing I could do about them. Being on an aeroplane that was banking and soaring in turbulence seemed outside my abilities, given I still felt dizzy on solid ground. Our whole family was state-bound because of me. I was tired of being the lowest common denominator that the family had to accommodate for.

After school, Jade boasted with excitement that her friend had seen the real Eiffel Tower in Paris. Now that she was older, she was seeking adventure and did not remember us taking her to Singapore as a baby. I wanted to share so many first travel experiences with her while choosing those she would most delight in. I wanted to watch her eyes widen as the plane took off into the clouds. I wanted to eat Nutella crepes with her at the little pop-up shop near the Eiffel Tower. We girls were gluttons for sugar. I wanted to feed crepe crumbs to the little sparrows under the table with her. She adored cute little creatures.

Tom and I had been to Paris during better times. What was once easily accessible to me was now under lock and key. Fear of missing out (FOMO) entered my life with a bang. Suddenly, I felt I was missing out on everything good in life. What started as FOMO of fine foods in restaurants now extended to travel.

Soon, FOMO was everywhere, even in our backyard. Tom assembled a trampoline as the most recent addition to our children's play equipment. Watching him jump up and down with them as they screamed with glee was bittersweet. I was happy they were happy, but I wanted to be part of that happiness, not watching from the kitchen window. They filled the enclosed trampoline with an assortment of balloons. As they jumped, the suspended colours transported the children to distant magical lands. On hot days, they hung misters on the trampoline, and the children played in their birthday suits, unabashed and uninhibited. They invented a game where they drew leprosy germs on a tennis ball that went up in random directions as they leapt, screaming, trying to get away from it. If all this fun was being had on a single trampoline, I did not dare imagine how much I was missing out on in the entire world.

I was still coughing and spluttering from the original cold I caught off Jade. I was convinced that I would have this cold for life. Viktor E. Frankl's words rolled around in my mind like thunderclaps rolled through the skies. In his book *Man's Search for Meaning*, he told the story of a fellow prisoner of war who had a vivid dream that he was to be released from the death camp on a particular date. When that date came and he was still in the same predicament, he died. Though he died of typhoid according to formal accounts, Viktor, a medical doctor and a professor of psychology and neurology, believed it was because he had given up hope. Hope is the vital ingredient for a fighting immune system. It had been over six months since I went deaf and became disorientated. I thought, *Perhaps I too have lost hope, and this cold is my typhoid.*

Chapter Nine

Mental Breakdown

The mind is its own place, and in it self
Can make a Heav'n of Hell, a Hell of Heav'n.
—*John Milton, poet*

Jade was trying to master dexterity, having recently transitioned from Duplo—the Jurassic version, designed for clumsy hands—to Lego. Her brows furrowed as she attempted to join two basic blocks together. Her shaky hands failed her a few times. When the joints clicked into place, she squealed with delight, proud of her accomplishment. I sat beside her, supervising her play. Jade's positive outlook regarding her underdeveloped coordination brought her hours of fun. It was unlikely that adults with Parkingson's disease would experience the same happiness with their trembling hands. The power of perspective was extraordinary. Maybe I too could come to terms with my limitations and even take joy from them.

The New Mother's Manual, if there was one, should come with a disclaimer that supervising children's play was only interesting for fifteen minutes before it became mind-numbing. I reached for my mobile and scrolled the newsfeed aimlessly.

BAM! Out of the blue, energy drained out of my body and into the earth. My arms fell to my sides, too weak to hold up my mobile. I slid down the wall I was sitting against. A cold flash came over me. My limbs and face tingled, and my heart raced. It felt like I was about to give a life-defining speech to a full auditorium. That or I was having a stroke. Just as I was about to pass out, I called for Tom. He rushed in at the urgency of my cry and helped me to the car.

I was still unconvinced that people just spontaneously became deaf and permanently woozy. I felt sure that whatever claimed my hearing half a year ago had come back for the rest of me. I was never sold on the diagnosis that I had a cold that went rogue. It all seemed a little hocus-pocus to me. I was doubtful that the worst was over.

But then the feeling of dread lifted while waiting in the emergency department. Energy returned to my arms and legs. Tom and I even had a pleasant conversation. The doctors took my vitals and ran my blood work to be sure before diagnosing what I'd had as a panic attack. I told them that was not possible. I had nothing to panic about. I was doing nothing at all when the alleged panic hit.

The doctor questioned if anything traumatic had happened to me recently. I told him about my ordeal with labyrinthitis.

"That will do it," he said. "You need to speak to a psychologist to help you grieve and reach acceptance of your prognosis."

There was that insinuation again, that I was in denial. Caring family, friends and well-intended doctors had been touting the need for acceptance as the remedy to my apparent denial for half a year now. Only there was nothing to deny. It was very clear that no sound was entering my left ear and that I was not steady on my feet. I fully understood what was happening to me. I was deaf and dizzy, not stupid.

I could only imagine how much more irritating this advice would be if I had lost a loved one instead. "Yes, I am fully aware he is dead. I was there when he turned blue and stopped breathing permanently," was a justification no one should have to make. I did not deny my fate. Rather, I was reconciling what was happening against the pre-existing narratives that I'd believed to be true. Those narratives had been formed based on my lived experiences before my life turned to custard.

Ironically, I was unfortunately blessed with parents who set me up with expectations of life that far exceeded what reality could deliver. My loving parents told me as a child that I could reach for the stars. Now, I could not reach for the overhead cupboards without risking a fall. Whenever I faced overwhelming challenges, they'd comforted me with "Don't worry, it's all going to work out in the end," and until now, that had been the truth. This time, the prognosis was definite. I would not be okay. Those pre-existing narratives had to be somehow reconciled with my current reality. My brain needed a coherent explanation before it could file this trauma away and begin forgetting about it. Since my worldviews did not seem to match up with reality, either what I believed to be true was a lie, or else this reality was not happening and I was going mad.

The writer Joanne Didion, in her memoir *The Year of Magical Thinking*, said it best when she discovered her husband's lifeless body on their living room floor. She described the scene as a rough draft, able to be rewritten before the story was finalised. That was how I felt. Something happened to me that was unthinkable and incomprehensible. My story needed to be rewritten because it made little sense, not because I could not accept it. Denial seemed an oversimplification of this process of making sense of the senseless.

I'd never once thought that being deaf and dizzy would be my story. That narrative never existed in my family's history. My grandparents collectively died from cancer, Alzheimer's, kidney failure, and a stroke. Being diagnosed with one of those would have made more sense, as if my ancestors were calling me to rejoin them at the family table. Instead, it appeared there had been a celestial clerical error, and they sent the rampant virus to the wrong address—my address. Surely, this was one big mistake that would rectify itself in time. It felt too surreal to be my reality.

Besides, I couldn't possibly have a panic attack because they were as real as Santa Claus. I had never subscribed to the whole mental health fanfare, nor had I experienced any of it myself. I once thought depression was just a label for sad people, anxiety was a clinical term for worrywarts, and panic attacks, well, they came from people having a bad day; nothing that couldn't be fixed by walking it off. R U OK Day was an annual event held on the second Thursday of every September in Australia that aimed to raise awareness about mental health and suicide prevention. As a senior manager, I wore the yellow T-shirts, walked around the department, and asked the right questions such as, "Are you okay?" I was respectful of mental health like I was respectful of religion: deep down, I never truly believed it was real. People making a big deal out of depression and anxiety to me was akin to the world making a big deal out of reindeer and sleighs every December.

Deaf. Dizzy. Endless vomiting. Getting my bottom wiped. Needle through the eardrum. Hyperbaric chamber. Walking frame. People staring. DING DING! "You fucking idiot!" Waking up in terror on repeat. Two university degrees and two decades of servitude, only to be left with a dying career. Just dying in general. Learning to walk and drive again. Jade not breathing. Failed hike. Unshakable colds. Barking mad canine. FOMO. Dashed dreams and a directionless future. All had culminated in this moment. The anxiety that was silently brewing had reached climatic proportions and erupted as a spectacular panic attack.

My initial panic attack opened a portal to mental health hell. I was now experiencing crippling anxiety daily, and if I could not talk myself off the metaphorical ledge, it would escalate to a full-blown panic attack. How I felt when I collapsed on the scratchy concrete pavement in the backyard, gasping for air to fill a pair of lungs that seemed to have sprung a leak, was more real than love. Depression, anxiety, and panic attacks were real, all right. They were invisible disabilities that I had been too naive to see or understand until now.

The decline in my mental well-being started around seven months after my trauma event. I did not know why it took so long to manifest but suspected it had something to do with permanency. At a subconscious level, I must have finally realised that my plight was here to stay. After trying everything I could with no success, I surrendered my fate to time but time did not heal all wounds like the adage said. The life I had planned, was looking forward to and counting on, was upended for real.

I had worked for two straight decades and felt run down from the throes of raising a young family, so there had been some relief in taking extended leave, labyrinthitis or not. But now it was no longer a holiday, albeit one that had been spent in hell. It was permanent. It was real, and it came at the expense of my future and livelihood.

Anxiety and panic ninjas tiptoed around in the shadows of my subconscious, sneaking up to hijack the controls of my body. I had another panic attack while soft-boiling an egg. Tom had to turn off the stove while I crawled to our bedroom. I couldn't hang in there long enough to see the egg through.

These attacks played out anytime and anywhere. While I was waiting in the drive-through line of Carl's Junior for our burgers. While supervising Jade play. While watering the garden in the sunshine. While shopping for groceries. While blow-drying my hair. While sipping a mug of hot chocolate. While lying in bed at night, doing nothing at all. And on it went. There were no threads of logic tying these attacks together. The feelings crept up and ambushed me.

It was impossible to fight an enemy in the shadows. The only defence I had was to breathe through it, four seconds in, four seconds out.

Anxiety became a self-fulfilling prophecy. The last time I tried to boil an egg, it failed spectacularly. I then felt too scared to boil another egg. When I pushed myself to do so, I became anxious about my anxiety. It reaffirmed I could no longer boil an egg, strengthening the negative feedback loop. I couldn't collect drive-through either. In fact, I couldn't do much of anything. My executive decision-making skill, which was my calling card, was replaced with analysis paralysis. I could not decide what I was going to do for the day. I was not sure what activities would make me hyperventilate.

My neurophysiotherapist was the fifth medical professional to suggest that I speak with a psychologist. He referred me to one who specialised in balance disorders. It surprised me that there was such a niche. My neurophysiotherapist explained he had spent a great deal of his career working in hospitals, rehabilitating patients from a wide range of circumstances. From what he had observed, patients who experienced vertigo were more troubled psychologically than any other patients. As a species, we crave the surety of outcomes, and unpredictability is bad for mental health. I could not trust the basic laws of physics, that gravity would do its job. Nor could I trust what I saw with my own two eyes. I was not spinning out of control, even though it felt like I was. I'd lost my anchor to reality and therefore my mind.

The fifth referral sat on my desk, piled up with the previous referrals. I wasn't ready to open Pandora's box to see how deep the rabbit hole went into something I'd only recently started believing in. Besides, I was sick of hanging out in doctors' waiting rooms. Already overwhelmed with managing my health, I did not want to add another loose thread to chase. I decided to leave my mind alone. To let it simmer and sort itself out.

Then an unexpected invite came to have lunch with a C-suite executive (let's refer to him as Peter for respectful anonymity). It was difficult to get an audience with him while I was actively working there, let alone after being missing in action for over half a year. He was a sought-after man. He packed his agenda back-to-back each time he flew to our state to squeeze every productive drop out of the visit. I was not sure to what I owed the pleasure of a one-to-one luncheon. The state of my mental health made me apprehensive about accepting his invitation. I did not have enough spine to sit through an entire lunch. Nevertheless, I clicked "Accept" on the invitation. Declining would be disrespectful to someone who had earned his way to that league and was giving up his time for me.

The venue nominated for lunch was in the building where I had worked. I would certainly run into several of my colleagues if not most of them. Employees transited through that building in droves during the busy lunch hour. Given that I abruptly pulled out of work and never returned, there was bound to be a stream of curious questions. I did not want to deal with answering them.

I got myself ready several hours before the luncheon, which gave me plenty of time to overthink and get myself worked up. This was a man I used to report budgets and unfavourable news to on a regular basis, but now I felt nervous having a panini with him. I reminisced about my fearless twenties, flying to England for the first time. After nearly thirty hours of travelling with no sleep, I'd hopped into a hire car and driven myself through peak London traffic in a city then unfamiliar to me. I did not feel a single knot in my stomach.

Now I was fearful of anything that moved, breathed, or even looked at me. I feared suffering, dying and never seeing my family again. I feared being anywhere outside of my home. Even my shadow had the jump on me. I was operating on the edge of anxiety and panic attacks. Anything requiring commitment from me, no matter how minuscule, tipped me over the edge, such as having friends over for dinner, being locked in a conversation with the neighbours, or leaving the house. How on earth was I going to cope with having lunch with a senior executive? I stood in front of the mirror and recited Shakespeare:

"Cowards die many times before their deaths. The valiant never taste of death but once."

Tom offered to take one stressor off the table by driving me into the city. Arriving at the venue, I chose a corner table close to the exit, facing the serving counter. Peter was late, which was not unusual, and understandable given his compressed schedule. Hungry patrons were queuing to order. Nothing about the scene was out of the ordinary until the man at the front of the line dropped his wallet to the floor. He then took off a shoe, revealing a sockless foot. In one seamless manoeuvre, he flicked open the wallet on the ground with his foot and pulled out a credit card between two toes. He did a controlled kick onto the counter, where the waitress took his card. I jumped back in my chair, startled. Really? After all that I had been through, I still reacted immaturely.

I now noticed that the arms of his suit jacket flapped around, empty of content. I had so many questions for him; most had to do with "How?" How did he type? How did he prepare a PowerPoint presentation? How did he come across to new customers? How was he going to eat his sandwich? Despite his challenges, he was getting on with business. The odds against him were worse than mine. I had worked for over a year in that building and I had never seen that man before. He must have been a regular here because the waitress didn't even flinch. Now I barely left the house and I got to cross paths with him.

That had to be more than happenstance. The universe was showing me willpower. It was telling me that dreams were possible regardless of circumstance. Initially frightened by the jarring truth I had witnessed, it ultimately schooled me. Where there's a will, there's a way.

Tom handed me off to Peter, who invited him to join us for lunch. Peter was in disbelief at what had happened to me—healthy and working for him one day, disabled the next. He wanted to see how I was doing and what I had planned moving forward. I had no genuine answers to his questions. I was still working things out for myself, and getting through to the end of the day was a major achievement at this point. Thank goodness a panic attack did not come on during lunch.

One of the key skills I was employed for was to see patterns in chaos and to bring about order. But I was at a loss as to what brought on the mental health episodes. It appeared to be random. It was an opponent I could not understand, which made it unbeatable.

The emergence of mental health issues wiped out the small gains I had made since I chose life. On the bright side, I appeared to have gotten over the cold I had been inoculating for months. It was as if the virus knew I had bigger fish to fry and that it was no longer a priority. I had my mental health to deal with now.

Chapter Ten

Self Worth

Success is to be measured not so much by the position that one has reached in life as by the obstacles which he has overcome.

—*Booker T. Washington, educator, author, and advisor*

My well-educated mum sacrificed her career as a Bank Manager for my sisters and me. Growing up, our family struggled financially, but we had a mum who nurtured and raised us closely. She told me often that I should never give up my livelihood for anyone, else I "would live under a man's thumb." She believed that dependency lent itself to abuse. She was my truth that kept me working hard.

I got my first professional salaried position when I left university and remained in the same company for just over twenty years. That was unheard of, especially with young graduates. Most of my colleagues company-hopped for pay rises. I didn't. I was focused on being excellent at my job and nothing else. A conqueror, I could never leave a job, person, or problem until I had it figured out. I needed to know how to run the organisation from the ground up and be capable of carrying out every role within my team. I wanted to be the teacher who could also do. Figuring out the total workings of a billion-dollar organisation was going to take a very long time, and I stayed to do so.

It turned out that the key to a stable rise in rank was to be good at your job. Networking and company-hopping got other people there faster, but without demonstrating consistent capabilities, the promotions stopped for them. I was one of the last people in my graduate cohort to excel, but over time, I surpassed the others. When I got offered promotions with more pay and prestige, it seemed illogical to turn them down.

I felt an overwhelming sense of gratitude towards my work. It had bought me my first car, my first home, and the lifestyle I was leading. I treated my job and company well, with respect and gratitude, like I would a person. I was good to the company, and she was good to me, especially when I needed her the most. I had squirrelled away a lot of sick leave over my many years of service, only ever using them for bedridden occasions. Financially, they honoured my sick leave for my extended time off with Labyrinthitis. They did not have to. I was not ill—I was disabled. Financially, it gave our family time to work things out. No one said or revealed anything to me, but in my heart, I know who the few people are who made this happen for me. Forever indebted. Forever grateful.

Mum brainstormed how else I could earn a living given my new limitations.

"You are always gardening—why can't you just grow a bit more and sell it?" Her proposals kept coming. She was more distressed about my career ending than I was. She had convinced herself that the loss of my career meant the loss of my independence and hence my freedom. However, the immediate loss I felt wasn't the pinch of decreased finances—it was the loss of my identity.

I had already experienced losing my identity since becoming a mum. With full-time work and two young children, there was no time to spend with friends, my tribe of the same feathers. A flamingo is surer that it is a flamingo when it looks around and sees other flamingos. I had forgotten how to be a friend. A lot of my hobbies also came to a halt when Jet and Jade were born. I used to get a buzz from taking raw ingredients and converting them into something useful: fabrics to dresses, seeds to gardens, alphabets to stories, and ingredients to cuisine. But I stopped being a creator because there was no energy left to create when the essential duties were done.

My identity had dwindled to being a worker and a mum. It pained me to admit that I was not maternal by nature. I performed the duties, but I didn't enjoy it enough to embrace my role as a mum. The sleepless nights, the messy play, and the unreasonable tantrums. In hindsight, it was because I never developed enough patience for it. I was the youngest of four growing up. I never had to baby anyone. They babied me. In my working life, I was surrounded by senior managers and intellectuals who operated at a high level. There was no opportunity to develop patience. Since Labyrinthitis took away my professional identity, being a quasi-mum was all I had left.

I considered all options to keep my career, but resignation was the wiser choice. My boss was exemplary in his support for me. He gave me a choice of any role that I could fulfil. This could mean working for one hour a week if that was all I could do. Despite this generous offer, I chose not to return to work for two reasons.

Returning to work would have rubbed the comparison in my face. By keeping every facet of my life exactly as before, I would know for certain that my life had got worse. I would lead the same life, but now as a disabled person. Returning to work would make the downhill trajectory obvious. Staying at home muddled the comparison. I could at least reason that I was no longer stuck in a small cubicle for most of the day. Instead, I was a disabled person who was spending time with my children soaking up the sunshine. There would be pros and cons to both, vastly different, lifestyles. The life before Labyrinthitis was apples and the life after was oranges. I could not directly compare the two. This, I am sure, kept away the last of the mental health trio, depression. I was already treading water dealing with anxiety and panic attacks. Adding depression by returning to work would have drowned me.

The other reason I chose not to return to work was because Tom and I had been in a deadlock since Jet was born. Our household fell into disarray, with two parents working full-time in demanding roles. The hours that were not spent working were spent on home chores. Shopping, cooking, cleaning, and laundry were the constant four. When Jade came along, our household became a Jenga tower on its last legs, wobbly and about to collapse.

Both Jet and Jade were high-needs children with unique challenges. Jet was now seven years old and had moved schools three times. That's once every year. The school year always started with optimistic teachers, confident in their abilities to tone down his big energy with regular breaks, fidget toys and wobbly cushions. By the end of the year, his teachers were glad to see the back of him. They firmly believed that Jet was autistic and pushed for medication. His paediatrician who specialised in assessing autism in children had assessed Jet as not autistic. Rather, Jet was a combination of highly intelligent, hyperactive, and defiant. The teachers rallied for a second opinion. I took Jet to the psychologist recommended by the school. On examining Jet, the psychologist came to the same conclusion. Jet was not autistic, rather he was hyperactive and lacked focus.

I dashed out from work every few days to listen as teachers vented about Jet's behavioural problems. Academically, he was ahead of the pack, which was an achievement, considering he had already skipped a year of school due to his high IQ. One night, he was in my arms for a quiet cuddle when he said, "Mummy, I know my brain is broken and I'm not like the others. That's why I get pulled out for special classes by myself." He was referring to the weekly sessions with the psychologist and the occupational therapist, which cost us thousands of dollars. It broke my heart to hear Jet say he was broken. That was the turning point when Tom and I decided to back our son and no one else. We chose not to medicate him and cancelled his rehabilitation. We were going to let him be himself. He had plenty of time to grow into his skin. If we had to deal with it at all, we could deal with it later.

People understand that different dog breeds need different environments. Sheepdogs need space to run out their enthusiasm, and Paris Hilton's dogs need designer handbags to snuggle in. Yet with children, the one-size school environment must fit all. Jet was not created to sit down indoors for six hours. The sheepdog in him wanted to roam, explore, work with his hands, and set things on fire. "Mum! Glass is made from sand. Can we go to the beach and collect sand to make some glass?" Jet would request.

As for Jade, her asthma was just the tip of the iceberg. When she was a toddler learning to walk, she fell and hit her head on the coffee table. The sound was louder than the bump. She cried briefly before stopping and turning blue as her eyes rolled to the back of her head. She convulsed. The seizure lasted a few minutes before her body went limp. She was still breathing, but her eyes were closed and she was unresponsive. Tom cradled her in his arms and said his goodbyes, thinking it was a brain bleed. I was hysterical, pacing around the house, screaming into the phone for an ambulance to come faster. They diagnosed her with Breath Holding Seizures. Whenever Jade was upset, scared, or angry, she would hold her breath, starving her body of oxygen with her iron will to the point of a hypoxic seizure.

She once experienced two seizures within a brief span of thirty minutes. She was sitting in her highchair having breakfast when she drifted off without a sound, convulsing. I thought she had choked and swept her mouth with my fingers. Little did I know, many fingers have been lost by doing this. People in the middle of seizures lock down their jaw at full force. I screamed in agony. Tom pried open her mouth to release my battered fingers. She was not choking. We must have fed her peas or broccoli, and she was not pleased. When the ambulance came, the paramedics took her from me. Her separation anxiety triggered another episode.

When she came to, she was not the same. She had regressed significantly. She could no longer walk, or talk, and wanted nothing more than to chew on my hair. It was as if Jade was missing a part of her brain. Our hearts were heavy, concerned we would not get our vibrant little girl back. Luckily, after several days, she healed completely from the oxygen deprivation. We were told that Jade would grow out of Breath Holding Seizures by six to eight years old. I heeded my uncle's warning that it was best to discipline her later rather than lose the chance to discipline her at all. Suffice it to say, we ended up raising a brat of a child who sometimes had chocolates for dinner.

One parent needed to be dedicated to keeping Jet and Jade alive. Tom and I had four degrees and bright futures between us. With comparable salaries, we were both hesitant to give up our careers, having come so far. In hindsight, this should have been a simple decision, but we were on a moving bullet train, and it felt difficult to hop off. The debate continued whether it was to be the house husband or housewife who made right our home.

Years passed in less-than-ideal settings. On the 8th of July 2021, the Universe decided for us and sent Labyrinthitis to my left ear. Life has a funny way of correcting its course. We knew what we should have done but didn't. Now it was done for us. It dealt me just the right amount of incapacitation, severe enough that returning to work was not an option, but sufficiently functional to run an effective household. I became a housewife, a position I never applied for. I decided I had better comply with the wishes of the Universe, or else it might smite me again.

Losing my livelihood had affected me more than I anticipated. The value a person contributes to society is easily quantifiable by their salary. That is how the world measures somebody's worth. Society rewards the worthy with access to the finest homes in prime locations, tables at the best restaurants, and cars that turn heads. It made sense to me to reward someone over another because they were more worthy. I had bought into this propaganda that my value was defined by how much I earned. A person was only valuable if they were productive in a way that could be compensated with money. The more compensation, the more the person was worth.

I ground up spices and toasted them in a pan over low heat. I was making Indian spinach and lamb curry from scratch. It took most of the day to make the curry and its many accompaniments. I watched Tom hoover down dinner with delight.

"Would you pay six hundred dollars for this meal?" I asked. Tom looked up warily, not sure where I was heading.

"Umm ... no?" he replied, possibly concerned I was going to charge for my labour at home.

"It took me a whole workday to make this meal. The same hands and brains made it. Mine. Shouldn't this meal be six hundred dollars?" I asked.

Unfortunately, it did not work that way. There was no causality between salary and a person's worth. Salary and perceived skills were positively correlated at best. My salary was determined based on what I was doing with my hands, brains, and skills and not on its virtues alone. It was not based on my capabilities, or how worthwhile the activity was. Rather, it was based on supply and demand. Many people could cook a mean lamb curry, but few could effectively run a Project Management Office.

Early in the Covid pandemic, Australia had defined a list of essential services. These were the work required to keep the country running, such as farming, grocery stores, sanitation, hospitals, and childcare for essential workers. Most of these were not high-paying jobs, relatively speaking. However, it had never been clearer that the people working to provide essential services were the ones doing the important jobs. After all, they had to keep working while the rest of us could stop. Their jobs were needed and mine was nice to have. I was now in an essential services role, providing childcare, albeit for my own children, and received no monetary compensation. Arguably, this was a more important job than what I had been employed to do. My worth was no longer defined by my salary. I had logically worked that out, but emotionally, my confidence took a detour to get there.

Shaken confidence in my social standing made me dissatisfied with what I had, leading me to reach for more—perhaps to convince others of my worth, or maybe to convince myself. Tom and I had always lived significantly below our means. Our values lay in gathering knowledge, not possessions. Our tiny home was in one of the poorest suburbs in the state. Jet once asked me while driving to school, "Mummy, why is that car propped up on bricks with no wheels?" I told him someone had stolen the wheels. Several days later, someone had graffitied the car and a few days after that, torched it. The kids were eager to see what else could happen to this poor car and rushed to get ready for school. One morning, the car was gone, removed by the council. Only the scorched bitumen remained.

We enrolled Jet into an elite private school far from where we lived. We were unwilling to compromise on a sound education. At school pickups, there was a battle over which mother had the better luxury SUV. I drove a modest car but did not mind. My quiet confidence could handle it. I knew our dual income could afford a pompous car if we wanted to, but Tom and I preferred to be sleepers, quietly successful without drawing attention.

However, my confidence waned when we were no longer humble by choice, dropping from dual to one income. It was easy to be silently smug about living poorly when I was only playing pretend. Tom could not understand my sudden frustrations with our living arrangements. We had been looking for more space to accommodate our growing family, but I was never motivated enough to get it done. It had always been a someday task that got pushed further out each time as that someday approached. I tried to articulate the change in feelings to Tom but could not do so successfully. I would have had to reveal my weakness, that I cared what people thought of me. Tom and I had always stood side by side in our belief that we ran our own race. I would be disappointing him if he realised I now felt differently. Tom was still sure of himself and his worth. I wasn't.

As we drove past the Aston Martin dealership, I tapped on my car window.

"Kids, look to the right, aren't those cars just beautiful? Pity I could never drive one now," I said. Jade questioned why. I explained I was not working anymore and therefore expensive luxury items were now out of reach for the foreseeable future.

"What can these cars do that others can't, Mummy? Why are they so expensive?" Jet asked.

"They drive like every other car, Jet, but only a few people can afford expensive things. It distinguishes them from the crowd. It's about social status. People see them with these cars and think, wow, they must be capable and amazing …" I trailed off at the absurdity of my explanation.

"Mummy, they are not amazing. They are dumb. For the same money they could get a car *and* a boat, and enjoy two different activities," Jet said matter-of-factly.

His refreshing point of view had not been tainted by the media, manufactured demands, or ego. He was right in every sense. I never aspired to luxury goods before and was not about to compensate now just because my self-worth and confidence took a beating.

It is hard to not waver when society repeatedly drums in that productive output defines the worth of a person. Even in extreme situations of life or death, hospitals triage who gets lifesaving help based on how many productive years they have remaining. I thought back to my diabetic friend in the hyperbaric chamber. I had told him how fortunate he was to be matched with a donor kidney as people tend to run out of life before that happens. The waitlist is painfully long because the system is predicated on someone dying before another can continue to live. Luck was not a factor, he explained to me. When his kidneys failed, he was young and considered the priority by the system. He pointed out that eventually his body would reject these kidneys because transplanted organs do not last a lifetime. He suspected they would give him another round of transplants and then deny him any further. Organs simply went to younger and more productive members of society.

Doors were opened to me before because I had ticked all the boxes of what it meant to be a highly productive member of society. Banks chased me down offering competitive loan rates, rival companies cold-called offering more pay, and strangers wanted to become friends. Now I did not tick any boxes, yet I remained the same person. Society needed to change its inaccurate definition of worth, instead of me lowering my worth to fit its unfeeling, narrow definition. Everyone will eventually retire to a less productive life. There is a guaranteed existential crisis waiting for everyone at the finish line. Mine got fast-tracked by a couple of decades is all.

The impermanence of form is a universal law, and I could accept that my body wasn't going to last forever. What I struggled with was the terrible timing of its breakdown. I felt robbed that my good times were cut short. People my age were supposed to be scuba diving, parasailing, and travelling the globe—not cooped up inside, sick. Each time someone asked, "Are you still deaf and dizzy?" I felt guilty for not measuring up to society's expectations, which were to heal. Young people were supposed to recover from illness, not remain ill indefinitely. Worse, I couldn't rest as one might expect a sick person to. I was not retired; my children had not left home. I couldn't curl up with a good book all day. I still had to put food on the table and my children through school, all while being sick.

Chapter Eleven

Existential Crisis

Don't try so much to form your character - it's like trying to pull open a tight, tender young rose. Live as you like best and your character will take care of itself.
—*Henry James, author and critic*

My worldviews were no longer bolted to the ground. So much of what I felt and believed with certainty was being challenged. Even my identity was in question.

My Human Resource lecturer for my post-graduate studies was a controversial sort. I never took a liking to him. He was passionate about analysing human behaviour and was convinced that common traits existed among all people. I distinctly remember him declaring smugly that non-disabled people were disgusted by disabled people. His allegation was met with beady eyes and pursed lips from his young audience. The concept of right or wrong was still black and white in our minds.

I recalled thinking, *No, you lunatic! I do not recoil when someone in a wheelchair pulls up beside me at the pedestrian crossing. If they need it, I will help them cross the road.* I dismissed what he was saying with little reflection. Yet his lectures stuck with me to this day, decades later, more so than any other lectures. Maybe it was the shock factor. Maybe the professor was being deliberately antagonistic. Or maybe these lectures held uncomfortable truths and I was once exactly as my lecturer described. I only came to defy his teachings because of my sister, who showed me a better way to be.

One school holiday, I'd travelled to Thailand and met up with my sister, Meena. She was seven years older than me and had been working abroad that year. Meena had acclimatised to their oppressive humidity, suffocating pollution and litter-lined roads. I, a mid-teen kid having just touched down from Australia, only knowing clear blue skies and sparkling beaches, experienced culture shock. It felt apocalyptic and I walked with my elbows tucked in, arms guarding my chest. Meena suggested we catch the bus for a day of shopping. The bus approached and slowed down, but never stopped. Meena shouted, "Jump in," and I followed her lead, untrained for this stunt. We sat down in the last two seats available, up at the front.

The bus slowed down at the next stop and a man hopped on who frightened me. He had long tendrils of soft flesh draping over his face that he parted to see where he was going. He looked like a character that Captain Jack Sparrow might encounter on the open seas rather than me on a midday bus in a bustling city. I remember thinking, *Thank goodness all the seats around me are taken. He cannot get close.* As he stood at the entrance of the bus fumbling for his coins, my sister spotted him. She sprang from her seat and made a beeline for him. She took his arm and escorted him to her seat, gesturing that it was now his. I sat with him the rest of the way, shoulder to shoulder, turning my head to look out the window. Not because I couldn't stand the sight of him; rather, I couldn't stand myself. I felt ashamed. It was a heavy lesson in humility. My sister, through her selfless example, showed me a higher moral code I could aspire towards.

"Why did you help him?" I asked upon leaving the bus.

"He needed it," Meena replied, her tone resolute that a person in need was enough of a reason to help. At that moment, my relationship with disability changed from a state of disgust to a state of sympathy. I felt people with disabilities were disadvantaged and extended a helping hand when the opportunity arose. My sister had helped me mature my views on disability part way. Navigating my trauma would mature my views the rest of the way.

Having lost a major sense and the ability to walk straight, the word "disabled" kept appearing in my consciousness, knocking on my door to have itself added to my identity. I was repulsed by that word being associated with me. *I am Nin the able, not Nin the disabled.* My lecturer was right. I still had a deep-seated prejudice against disability that I was not aware of. Disability was good enough for others, but not good enough for me.

I cringed at the thought of disability being added to my identity because it felt like I would be a lesser person. That was prejudice. Passing comments such as "Are you deaf?" that went unnoticed before now had my attention, as if someone had called my name. Even though the question was rhetorical, an answer always sprung to mind: "Yes, I am." I am now mindful to never use lines like "Are you blind?" or "Are you senile?" You may think me too sensitive and politically correct. Rather, I prefer to think that I had joined a small club of people in the know and that if I had become anything, it was less naive.

I questioned what else I was prejudiced about. My closest friends were all from different cultural backgrounds, and I loved that. Our dinner parties looked like a *United Colours of Benetton* ad. We conversed from different perspectives and our healthy debates piqued my interest. If I woke up suddenly Italian or Vietnamese, I hope I would be okay with that, and that it was not a case of other races being good enough for my friends but not for me. Obesity. LGBT. Poverty. I had friends spanning all groups. The thought that I might have felt contempt for them at any level like I did for disability made me uncomfortable. It appeared I had prejudices to confront that lay buried deep and dormant.

I had to work through many new labels. "Unemployed" was another. With Jet changing schools like they were socks, I got to meet many new people. They were mainly the parents of Jet's newfound friends. The polite greetings rarely lasted longer than a few minutes before the question of what I did for a living came up. It had been a straightforward question to answer when I was an engineer, a project manager, or an executive. Since I had stopped working, I could never answer without feeling awkward. I knew my place in society as measured against the salary yardstick.

"I'm currently not doing anything," I would say with a weak smile, avoiding using the word "unemployed."

Right on cue, they would follow up with "Oh, just taking a break from work?"

Nine times out of ten, a simple "Hello" would lead to me handing over my health history to strangers. That made the conversation even more uncomfortable as people grappled with what to say in response to my disability.

No one ever asked, "How is your son settling into the new school?" People were interested in my occupation as a criterion to assess our potential friendship as if to rule out prostitution, drug mule, and crime boss. Sometimes I would say, "I'm just at home looking after my kids." The "just" always appeared in that sentence. Their responses were predictable. "Raising children is one of, if not the most important jobs." Yeah, nah. I doubt anyone truly believed that. Me before Labyrinthitis didn't.

Now, I never ask people what they do for a living, especially at the first meeting.

Labyrinthitis had split my identity and timeline into two: me before it, and me after it. I could vividly remember the weekend before the illness. Tom was on a ladder, picking olives from the neighbour's tree that overhung its branches into our yard. I was sitting under the back veranda with Jet and Jade, pitting olives and getting them ready for pickling. I couldn't tell you what I was doing the weekend before that and beyond. My mind only took a snapshot of the moment right before everything changed and etched it into my memory.

Before my health trauma, I was a proud lioness prowling the land, capable of the hunt. The me after was a scared little rabbit, cowering in a shadowy corner of the room. Instead of my life being one continuous storybook, there was now a sequel with a clear break in between the volumes. Who I was as a character in the first book of the two-part series was clear. Who I was in the sequel was still being developed. I couldn't even decide on what to wear and hadn't a clue whether to buy the dress on the rack. I wasn't working anymore and could venture beyond the professionalisms of navy, black and beige, but colours were confronting and I was no clown. At every turn I froze with inaction because I could not answer the author and businessman Seth Godin's question, "Do people like us do things like this?" This question allegedly drove people's decision to act. I didn't know my identity, let alone the group I should be a part of. If I could see people like me doing things like this, then I would do it. But who was like me? I was paralysed with inaction.

The trained engineer in me began to parameterise the problem, breaking it down into simpler, more solvable chunks.

Surely what defined a person couldn't be as shallow as what they wore and owned, though that could provide a clue. Perhaps dressing modestly meant the person was conservative, for instance. We could say the same about the company they kept. These were all breadcrumbs leading back to someone's identity. And if actions spoke louder than words, then what defined a person ought to be the sum of their actions that led to their current station in life. Their achievements mattered in forming an identity. After all, grit, discipline, and ambition were all facets of identity synonymous with great achievements. I had no idea where kind-hearted, loyal, and cheery dispositions fitted into the puzzle, but I am sure they had pieces in the box. Maybe we ought to examine a person's occupation as they spent a lot of their time doing it. Given that most people spent their work week counting down to the weekends, day jobs done under duress weren't an accurate reflection of someone's identity.

If people would rather pursue their hobbies and interests, then perhaps their passion projects could reveal their identity. However, jobs, hobbies, and interests were all centric around what a person could do. I could no longer do what I did, but surely my ear and its inner workings didn't define me. Consider the case of an elite athlete who lost their mobility. Were they still an athlete? Was a mother whose child had passed still a mother? The answer felt like it had to come from within. Identity seemed intrinsic to a person. It should be impossible, or at least difficult, to separate the person from their identity. An accident that rendered the athlete immobile could not take away his drive and commitment. The sickness that claimed the child could not change the heart of his mother, forever nurturing and selfless. But women weren't born mothers; they started as babies and became little girls. Identity appeared to have an ever-changing baseline. The concept blew around in the wind of new experiences and reflections. Race, gender, religion, nationality, age, health, wealth, education, skills, achievements, intelligence, temperament, personality, demeanour, virtue, jobs, hobbies, tastes, rationales, friends, addictions, relationships, and roles. It's no wonder many people struggled to find themselves. If identity was fickle, then it could not have been that important to begin with.

My sister Nan and I shared a room until we were teenagers. Surely she knew the real me. Nan knew I was obsessed with cleanliness. She could get me to cry by touching me with a broom, and not even the dirty end. I should ask her who I was.

"I don't know who I am anymore!" I cried.

"You are who you have always been: my little big sister. The person who makes all the right decisions. The person I come to for advice. You have always been the person who is organised and has it together. The smart and sensible one amongst us," she said.

To her, my identity was not what I did, but how I did it. I was sensible in any situation and thought matters through. Logical, risk averse, task driven, and well planned. I was not very spontaneous (to Tom's dismay), especially on holidays. I would book restaurants in advance for all three meals during the entire vacation. Tom would rather select his meals by wandering down strange alleys and having a little neon sign catch his eye. Marriage was about compromise, so I planned in spontaneous hours in the holiday schedule just for him. He got to decide on a whim how we were to spend the allocated spontaneous slot.

Pinning down an accurate description of identity when the inputs kept changing was like playing a game of whack-a-mole. I was already struggling to understand who I was since becoming a mum; add disability into the mix and I did not know whether I was Arthur or Martha. There were too many contributions, several of which were not static. Even the steadfast parts of my identity—a daughter, sister, mum, and wife—were not strong enough to maintain their ground. A dramatic change in my health status was enough to cause an identity crisis.

My children were never one to sugarcoat the truth, not even to spare feelings. One time, we were leaving *K-Mart* when I asked Jet to "Show the nice lady our receipt."

"That's a man! That is definitely a man!" Jet protested, pointing his finger to make sure I knew exactly who he was talking about. If I could go back in time, I would have left it there. Instead, I corrected him. That poor well-built woman.

Right now, I needed their honesty to help resolve who I was and called Jet and Jade into the room.

"Jet, who are you?" I asked.

"A kid," Jet answered without hesitation.

"What about you, Jade? Who are you?"

"A girl," Jade replied in a flash.

Simple but not confused. It need not get more complicated than that. I was an adult, having adult experiences and getting through them based on how I felt at that moment. I didn't need to ponder my identity at all. I was uncertain of myself as a teenager, as a young adult, as a professional, as a working mum and now as a less able, unemployed person. The same uncertainty awaited when our children moved out of home or when we retired. The effort to redefine my identity was not worth the confusion and headache. I did not need to identify any factors besides my name that distinguished me from other people. Identity was the basis of comparison and division, not conducive to the establishment of common ground. The ego was an impossible master to appease. It was time to walk away. As an identity, just being an adult was enough for me. I was released from the social expectations associated with a defined version of myself. I just needed to confirm that Tom didn't miss her too much.

When I first met Tom, he described my character as "A happy yappy little dog that rushes up to greet every passerby at the fence, tail wagging madly."

I had not smiled in months, at least not genuinely. I wondered how Tom felt about the woman he married, whether he still saw me in the same endearing light. We conversed long into the night about it. He said that from his point of view, nothing had changed except that our household ran better with me at home.

I pressed on, getting past the logistics and onto how he really felt about his wife, whether I was still happy and yappy. Tom confessed that he too had to mourn the loss of my physicality. He used to have a robust companion that he could rumble and tumble with and literally sweep her off her feet. He missed me lying in his arms in bed, turning freely to meet his gaze. His wife had been replaced with a delicate vase that he had to handle with care at all times, or risk breaking. He mourned the death of tickling, play roughhousing, and dancing in our living room. Invisible disability came with no warning labels; for the most part, I looked fine. The mental load was on him to live cautiously and handle me gently.

Tom smirked to lighten the atmosphere. "It's not all bad. To be honest, I was sick of living under the tyranny of Hearing Nin. Deaf Nin is much kinder and more understanding. There is something beautiful about vulnerability."

Indeed, many a true word is spoken in jest. Before I was befallen, there was an arrogance that came with believing myself invincible. It was easy to be brave and confident when I thought of myself as an immortal. I had minimal understanding of the human struggle because life had dealt me too many aces. It wasn't until I fought through my own struggles that I found true humility.

There is no act humbler than accepting help.

Previously, I was too arrogant to accept help because I was above handouts. I wore my independence with pride, like a badge of honour, believing that there was nothing I couldn't achieve with my own two hands. Believing that I did not need anyone for my happiness or survival. I even justified this viewpoint in our marriage. Matrimony is the ultimate symbol of intertwining lives, but I explained to Tom that when two wholesome people came together, who did not need one another but wanted to be with each other by choice, that was the real deal. On reflection, perhaps I was fiercely independent because I did not have the patience for people, in much the same way I did not have the patience to raise my children.

Getting my bottom wiped made me realise that I was not always going to be a pillar of strength. There would be moments when I needed to lean on others and them on me. I thought of my mum's warning that total dependence was a weakness for others to exploit. However, my trauma had taught me differently: that the sweet spot was somewhere in between dire dependency and the lone wolf I had been.

I had witnessed the delicate and beautiful dance of give and take, and it surpassed any solo performance I could have choreographed. Regardless of how independent I perceived myself to be, I existed as part of the interconnected paradigm of nature. An ancient proverb states, "Nothing in nature lives for itself. Rivers don't drink their own water. Trees don't eat their own fruit. Sun doesn't give heat for itself. Flowers don't spread fragrance for themselves."

I fell in love with the idea of communities and began reaching out to neighbours that I had never known. They extended back, and we became a community.

Margaret Mead, an American Cultural Anthropologist, was asked by a student what the first sign of civilization was. She replied that civilization began when there was evidence of a healed femur, the thigh bone. She reasoned that animals suffering from significant injuries like this would die from starvation or be eaten before they had the chance to heal. To have a femur healed meant that someone had taken care of the injured, nursing them back to health. The emergence of human civilization was without a doubt the most significant milestone in human history. Without civilization, I would still be collecting berries and Tom spearing fish.

Nurturing the positive evolution of society became important to me. Previously, I couldn't understand the magic of give and take. I only understood how to give. Without the take, it made others feel small whilst I alone felt big. I no longer aspired to be the smartest person, the richest person, the most righteous person or the most anything person. I wanted to become the person who was conducive to creating a wholesome society.

Had I been religious, I would have asked myself what Jesus would do. Instead, before an action, I would ask whether it was helping or hindering society in the greater sense. I did a little exercise to make sure I understood what I was thinking. Raising children to become wholesome adults: helping. Creating technology that connected people: helping. Creating addictive technology that turned people into zombies: hindering.

This lone wolf was now part of the pack.

Chapter Twelve

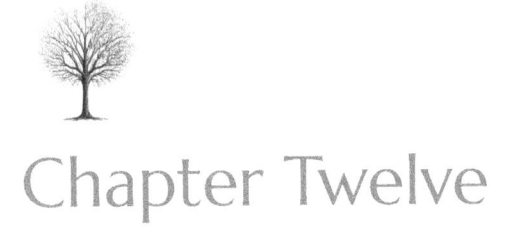

Facing the Demon

To keep the body in good health is a duty... otherwise we shall not be able to keep our mind strong and clear.
—*Siddhartha Gautama, Buddha*

A few years earlier, one evening after the kids had gone to bed, there had been a knock at the door. It was not uncommon to get a police visit late in the night, living where we lived. Tom answered the door. It was his close mate, showing up unannounced with a bottle of whiskey, the kind where no expense was spared. They went to the backyard, drank, and laughed together. When his mate left, both men were grinning ear to ear.

Tom looked surprised, like when a child spoke a sentence before they managed a first word. "Wow, that was nice of him," I remember saying as we settled back into our snuggle and Netflix. A few days later, our mate was unreachable. We called, messaged, and e-mailed. Eventually, a dreaded response came from a mutual friend. Our close mate had taken his own life. He had battled with anxiety and depression on and off since we had known him. He had lost the fight against his demons. What ultimately caused his demise were the same drugs that were saving him; he had just taken too much. Our friend's case had formed our views on drugs for treating mental illness. Tom and I learnt that having such powerful state-altering drugs on hand, at the ready, was not always a good idea, especially when one was desperate to change their feelings. It only took a moment of instability to go overboard with medication. Tom and I never wanted to lose one another. We agreed we were going to remedy the pressures of life with healthy habits instead. Medication was to be the last resort.

Jade was only a few months old when Tom's demons showed up. There was no noticeable trigger. I suspected it had to do with a man loving his wife, his wife loving their children, and no one to love the man. The Covid pandemic exacerbated the situation, bringing stagnancy to life and business, robbing Tom of his passion for progress. I had dramatically less time for Tom when Jet was a toddler and Jade was a baby. They were both attached to me and wanted no one else. I couldn't support him as I had no capacity to do so. Worse, I did not understand what he was going through. Tom was incapacitated, with no official diagnosis. He lost his appetite and had to be coerced to eat the meals that usually he would enjoy. The gruelling days frustrated me because I was without my partner, my rock. Jet and Jade were screaming, and I was rushing to them in different rooms.

"Get rid of it! Whatever you are feeling, get over it. There are children that need attending to! They are real and will die if we don't feed them. They don't exist in your imagination like whatever you have. Get rid of it!" I ordered.

Tom's demeanour shifted from despondent to alert, as if he had been jolted out of his apathy. The intensity of my command overrode his internal turmoil, at least in that moment. I must have been a monster more fearsome than what he was fighting with. Though effective, it wasn't right and far from my proudest moment. I didn't support Tom with what he went through. Both of us were overwhelmed, I with our young children and he with his mind. We could not be there for one another. He had to navigate his depressive terrain alone, emerging victorious on top of the mountain he climbed with his own two legs. When my demons showed up, Tom was experienced and stood strong beside me. World-class hugs, celebrating reaching the end of the day, boxes of chocolates and listening without judgement. He did it all.

After several months of debilitating anxiety and panic attacks, I learnt to fight back against my opponent, landing a few jabs of my own. I expanded my tool kit beyond regulated breathing and could now recognise the early warning signs. Symptoms were many: lightheadedness, weakness throughout the body, cold flashes, tingling face, derealization, and stomach churns, to name a few. I had come to know anxiety rising as an overall feeling. "I feel like a wisp," I would say. For those unfamiliar with fantasy realms, let me get some geek out of the way. A wisp is a delicate supernatural creature depicted as a small ball of glowing light, floating ethereally. Except I had no magical powers. I had no power to even stand on my own two feet.

I discovered by chance that when I changed the state of my body with big movements or a temperature change, the wispy feeling stayed at bay and never eventuated to a panic attack. My goal was to avoid anxiety escalating into a panic attack at all costs. Teetering at the edge of a cliff, though scary, was far better than falling off. Panic attacks were torture in a different league. I would collapse into a pile of laundry, vomiting. To stop the escalation, the moment I felt anxiety rising, I shifted the state of my body. If I was sitting, I would stand and do power poses borrowed from Wonder Woman. If I was rugged up and cosy, I would splash cold water on my face. By pulling the rug from underneath the anxious bodily state I was in, I could disarm the panic attacks before they escalated.

I wanted the anxiety to stop altogether, to never experience being a wisp again. I wanted to find the root cause that was triggering my anxiety. Our bodies run on sophisticated software, albeit the organic version that uses hormones instead of variables. They don't behave randomly. Given that I'd had anxiety in almost every scenario, my body was responding to inputs that were eluding me. While I didn't know my enemy, I could work on my armour and defence. I had become a fearful person, and I didn't like it. I needed to work on my bravery first.

I had never understood the point of listening to positive affirmations. It had no logical basis. Hearing that I was beautiful didn't change my appearance or the beauty standards of society. Sure, if I heard it often enough, I could come to believe it. If that were the case, I would be delusional because the tangible truths never changed. However, belief was enough for a desperate situation. I needed to believe that I was brave, the world was safe, and there was nothing to fear. YouTube had a robust catalogue of healing and health-related affirmations.

"My immune system is healing my body. My health is getting better each day. My body is strong and resilient," played on the speakers.

I was astounded at how well these affirmations worked. I started to believe that my body was a well-engineered machine I could trust and delegate the healing efforts to. Once delegated, it was a slight weight off my shoulders. Positive affirmations were like vitamins, I discovered. A healthy body would get rid of extra vitamins as waste. A healthy and resilient mind got rid of positive affirmations with cringeworthy disregard. My broken mind was soaking up these affirmations like cracked earth absorbing torrential rain.

"If they didn't work, love, people wouldn't be creating so many of them," Tom said, smirking at my closed mind being blown to bits.

When Tom and I were building a fence for our house, we noticed fences everywhere, having never paid attention to them before. Our minds were programmed to focus on fences. I could only describe houses we passed by in terms of pillars, spears and COLORBOND finishes. My medical trauma had programmed my mind to focus on danger cues. I was hyper-attuned to things that could harm or kill me, and they existed in abundance. I was living in survival mode, in a fight-or-flight state.

To counter my fears, I spent the day seeking safety cues instead. Here is what I noticed. Medical centres were plentiful, scattered every few blocks. Doctors were close by, as were medicines. There were no shortages of pharmacies. Adults walked the streets who could seek help on my behalf. The roads were full of drivers who could get me from A to B fast. I often spotted ambulances and police cars among the traffic. My mobile was well charged and in my pocket. Tom and Mum were on speed dial. They were never more than a twenty-minute drive away. Our city wasn't big. I was going to be okay until help arrived, and if I wasn't, I wouldn't have suffered for long. I repeated the exercise of searching for safety over many days until the world was no longer an active threat. The erratic mouse darting back and forth in my head could now sit still and enjoy some cheese.

Growing up, I recalled my parents being anxious the moment we pulled out onto the street in our car. They would start running through whether they had locked the doors and turned off the stove. This was a few minutes after they had physically done the inspection rounds. We lived in a rough neighbourhood and they had no rainy-day funds, so I understood the importance of not stuffing up. Small oversights had big consequences for a family living bare-bones. Their thoughts triggered their anxiety, compounding their worries. It appeared to be happening in their conscious mind. My anxiety was different. It bypassed my conscious mind altogether.

The subconscious mind must have been a woman. It made the conscious mind believe it was in charge, pacifying its big ego while pulling the strings in the background. I had a glimpse into how powerful it was when I learned after a few months of waking up in vertigo hell to keep my body still. I was no longer moving in my sleep and got the eight hours of rest I needed. Whatever position I fell asleep in, I would wake in that position. I had a bit of fun with it, crossing my arms over my chest and falling asleep like The Count in a narrow tomb. When I woke, I was still posed as Dracula. The first movements were the hardest, akin to the liquid nitrogen scene in Terminator II. My joints locked up and my bones ached. I felt like the stiff undead, but I wasn't complaining. Solid sleep was the turning point in my recovery. Time healed trauma in an unexpected way. Despite still being deaf and dizzy, my suffering reduced as I tore off days from the calendar. I was now sleeping.

My bread-and-butter skill was taking disparate data and turning it into usable knowledge. After upwards of twenty panic attacks and even more anxious days, I had enough data points for a trend to emerge. I knew that panic attacks were triggered when I felt a change in bodily sensation. Hungry, tired, thirsty, full, hot, cold, sleepy, achy, excited, and bored. There were many sensation changes throughout the day, but not all of them made me anxious. Pareto principle taught me that eighty per cent of outcomes resulted from twenty per cent of causes. That meant most of my panic attacks were triggered by a few sensation changes. I was close to nailing the sucker down.

I swiped the entire section of books relating to anxiety into my online trolley. Through these books, I learnt that anxiety originates in two pathways. The first is the cortex, which is the thinking and reasoning part of the brain. I had been referring to it as the conscious mind up to this point. Thoughts originating in the cortex can trigger anxiety, such as my parents second-guessing obsessively whether the stove had been turned off. Most therapies treat the cortex pathways by working to change thoughts and perceptions. I was doing exactly that when I spent my days looking for safety cues.

The second anxiety pathway is through the amygdala, which I had been referring to as my subconscious brain. The amygdala, also known as the "reptilian brain" or the "primitive brain", is small but a force to be reckoned with. It processes emotions, particularly fear and pleasure. The amygdala attaches these emotions to experiences, forming emotional memories. In high-stress, risky situations where a split-second decision is required, the amygdala takes over. Encountering a stimulus that is attached to an emotional memory, especially one that is identified as a threat, will trigger fear. The fear response sets off anxiety, placing the body in survival mode. The amygdala can hijack the decision-making, bypassing the rational, higher-order brain altogether. My reading cemented my vague suspicions of what was happening to me. I needed to identify the stimuli that were setting off my fear response and consequently my anxiety and panic attacks.

In her book titled *Rewire Your Anxious Brain*, Dr. Pittman describes how, when the senses receive information that is reminiscent of a traumatic emotional memory, the amygdala initiates an anxiety response. She cites a curious case of a grown man panicking whenever he saw a teddy bear. His amygdala interpreted the teddy as a threat. When he was a little boy, his grandma held out a teddy bear as he ran towards her. He fell over, sustaining significant injuries to his face. His conscious brain did not remember this incident, but his subconscious brain did.

Another intriguing case was a war veteran who had returned home from service. He was assimilating well back into society when panic attacks started occurring daily. There were no obvious triggers at first, but through investigations, he realised that his wife had changed his soap. The scent of the new soap was the same scent he'd used when stationed in combat. He got rid of the soap and his anxiety disappeared.

I thought back to my trauma event. It wasn't difficult to recollect, as it was the only tragedy that had overwhelmed my ability to cope. That tragedy had been filed away as a threat by the amygdala. I conjured up in my mind's eye the day I was wheeled off on a stretcher to the emergency room. I tried to remember the predominant feelings and sensory inputs during that day and week. Ears ringing and violent vertigo. After my trauma, if I was experiencing vertigo, or if my healthy ear experienced ringing, it was a given that I could count on a panic attack for sure. I expected that. It would be a reasonable natural response. I would know there was a logical basis to it, and that I wasn't going insane. Rather, it was the spontaneous anxiety and panic attacks for no apparent reason that made getting through the day difficult. I needed to find the reason for these.

Then it came to me. On the night of my traumatic experience, I was busting to pee and felt unbearably hot and sweaty. I then spent the next five days unable to move, staring up at the white ceiling, feeling mind-numbingly bored. For me, those three sensation changes explained almost all onsets of my random anxiety.

My body temperature rose while I blow-dried my hair, sipped on a mug of hot chocolate, or watered the garden in the sunshine. That was enough for the amygdala to start its threat sequence. Those sweatpants were still terrorising me. Needing to empty my bladder explained my panic attacks while watching a movie and I was too lazy to get up, and the time I was shopping for groceries and couldn't abandon my trolley. Boredom was the biggest culprit. Each time my mind wandered while supervising my children play, boiling an egg, going to bed when I wanted to stay up, or waiting around for drive-through, I would pay for it. I had identified my triggers, but how was I going to manage them? Cues to empty my bladder, fluctuations in body temperature and an idle state of mind were normal functions of human biology. They were built-in features that I couldn't discard like the Sergeant did his soap.

I put workarounds in place. To avoid a full bladder, I would excuse myself to the ladies far ahead of needing to go. Some hours I returned there twice, just in case. To ensure I didn't get too hot, I would spritz myself with cold water before stepping out of the shower and finish my hair styling with the dryer set to cool. And as for boredom, I would set the egg timer and walk away. While the kids were climbing and sliding in the playground, I used the nearby trail to get my daily step count up to ten thousand. Sitting on the park bench staring out into space was what the amygdala was scanning for. I wasn't going to give it the satisfaction.

Through diligent management of triggers, spontaneous anxiety and panic attacks dropped from several times a week to several times a year.

Neuro-links had formed between my triggers and seeing them as threats. I wanted these connections in my brain obliterated. Not worked around or managed, but destroyed. A terrible experience had scrambled my mind and neuroplasticity was going to train my brain out of it. My three troublesome sensations and I were going to become friends. I extended the olive branch by allowing myself to be with these sensations until anxiety showed up. I sat wriggling and squirming as my demon rose, taking on a hazy form. Before it could grow powerful enough to do actual damage, I would release the triggering sensations by cooling down, relieving my bladder, or breaking the monotony. My demon dispersed like grey smoke in the breeze. My body relearnt that no harm came with these sensations, and soon I could endure them in larger doses. Unbeknownst to me, what I had done was a therapy technique called habitualisation. As these new safety connections strengthened, the threat link that had formed during my trauma weakened, but never severed. I was no longer anxiety's bitch, and it was liberating.

This process took a gruelling nine months before I got my anxiety and panic attacks under control to the point of being able to function daily. In hindsight, my triggers are rather obvious. This is not the case for everyone. I am aware there are others still figuring out their triggers, possibly even after a lifetime of anxiety. With no intention of belittling anyone else's struggles and experiences, I only share mine to provide hope that it's possible to vanquish your demons.

Chapter Thirteen

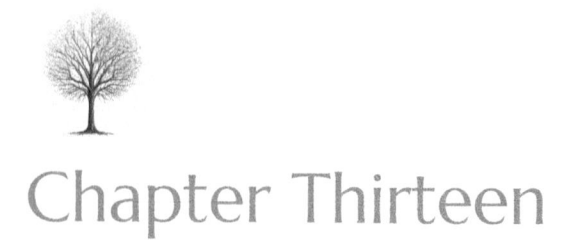

Unhappy Anniversary

There is no grief which time does not lessen and soften.
— *Marcus Tullius Cicero, statesman, orator, and author*

Anniversaries differ from other days. They mark a place in time. Anniversaries used to be joyous occasions that came with a generous spread of food and alcohol. The anniversary of my birth, the birth of my children, Christmas, New Year, and, of course, my wedding anniversary to Tom. The 8th of July, however, was not one of those.

I could see the date creeping in from a distance. It marked the unhappy anniversary of my downfall. That date took the life I loved, chewed it up and spat back out something unrecognisable. It was the day I took a tumble and never stood back upright. That dreaded date will forever be remembered. I even recall the moment the shit-show started, right down to the minute.

Upon returning home from the hospital, family and friends dropped by my house to offer their initial sympathies and never returned. Why should they? It wasn't a fun encounter. Awkward at best. People were at a loss for what to say to me. Most told me it was going to be okay, not knowing that it would. I had a few curious questions about my condition that were facepalm worthy.

"Can you still talk normally, or do you now speak like deaf people?" a friend asked.

"I wasn't born deaf!" I replied. "I learnt to talk normally like you did."

I needed a friend to sit with me through my grief and not have it define my interactions with them. I didn't want to be told I would recover when I knew it was a lie. I didn't want to answer any more oddball questions either. People tried to relate by telling me about their bad days. I would take anyone's bad day over mine. Car troubles? No worries. Didn't get that promotion? Try again.

Around two months after I got struck down, it was my birthday. If anyone asked, I would deny it, but as the day approached, a small part of me was hoping for a miracle on my special day. I would wake in the morning to find balloons in the living room, the children shouting with glee, and that this nightmare was just a product of my sleep deprived imagination. Wouldn't that be nice? Yet the realist in me was sure my birthday was going to be tainted with sorrow, and I was not looking forward to it.

My phone chirped. A dear friend invited me to my favourite restaurant in a quaint countryside town for paella and sangria. She knew the combination of my two loves, sensational food and greenery, was the cheese needed to lure this meek mouse out of hiding. I agreed to go, not knowing if I could last the entire outing. It was early days since the ordeal, and my head still felt like it was riding waves in rough seas. She had booked a table and invited our mutual friend and her family to join us. She organised flowers and a cake. Three families with a few festive touches turned an ordinary lunch into an intimate party. Tom set the tone by speaking painfully slowly, exaggerating his pronunciation with his lips, directing me to "Paaaass thhhhee saaaaalt pleeeaase," emphasizing my hearing issues. I shot him a dirty look, and the table roared with laughter. The message was clear: let's have some fun today. And we did. My birthday was fantastic.

However, my birthday failed to deliver the results I was hoping for; still deaf and dizzy. So did Christmas and New Year.

The 8th of July was nothing like my birthday. Leading up to my unhappy anniversary, I felt like a sheep tagged with bright blue paint, destined for the abattoir. I did not want this date to happen. The logical part of me knew that it was just another day. However, my emotional side brewed up a dark thunderstorm. I spent the day reflecting on my ordeal, the unfairness of it all and how hard my life had become. I felt sorry for myself and cried whenever no one was watching. Being taken out of the scene for one year was a sabbatical. Any longer was a lifestyle. It was common for people to take a year off work and embark on a self-discovery journey. My anniversary informed me that this wasn't that. This was permanent, my new undesirable norm. Acceptance took many bites of the cherry, asking a bit more of me whenever it had the chance. I was glad to be rid of the day.

People were still asking me after a year whether my hearing had returned and if I was still dizzy. I would reiterate the fact that I had a permanent disability. I explained that the organs responsible for hearing and balance were destroyed; not a little bit, but a total write-off. Still, people kept asking about improvements to my condition. I wondered whether amputees had similar questions asked of them. "Have your limbs grown back yet?" Perhaps the scepticism was only around invisible disability because it did not come across as real enough. Or perhaps good news made everyone feel better and people were on the constant lookout for it.

After three hundred and sixty-five days of waking up unsteadily, I stopped mentioning these unpleasant sensations altogether, even to Tom. Talking about it had become as tedious as a conversation about the weather, especially for the listener. Complaining never eased my symptoms anyway. I sucked it up and dealt with the discomfort in silence. Lo and behold, when I stopped whining about it, people stopped asking me if my incurable disability had gone away. It was me all along who was soliciting those absurd questions. A year was long enough for me to stop updating people on these same feelings. Uncomfortable every day was the new status quo. Much like feeling hungry, people didn't complain when their stomachs rumbled. They just dealt with it.

On the anniversary of my illness, it became clear that I was playing the long game. It reminded me of a popular metaphor for stress, where a teacher requests a student to hold up a glass of water and asks whether it feels heavy. The student replies that it does not. After half an hour, the teacher asks the student again. That same glass of water now feels like lead. Carrying a chronic illness is a similar experience. I would walk on burning coals if there was an end in sight. The human spirit can bear any level of pain if there is an exit. The long game was different. The long game required sheer tenacity beyond anything that had ever been expected of me before. I became jealous of anyone with acute temporary problems, no matter how severe.

I envied people getting divorced. As I listened to my friend pour his heart out about how his wife packed up and left him without warning, I kept thinking that he would find someone else in time, and none of this would matter. Sure enough, he started dating again. Another friend had a stroke which temporarily paralysed half of his body. After a couple of months, he made a full recovery. Lucky him, I thought. Why couldn't I have had that stroke instead? I wanted to be dealing with a temporary problem. I was miserable at being the only person I knew with permanent loss and everlasting challenges to deal with. Rightly or wrongly, everyone else's problems became trivial compared to mine because they were short-lived.

There was an upside to my unhappy anniversary. It meant that enough time had passed for memories to fade. I couldn't tell you what hearing in stereo sounded like anymore. In theory, I knew it sounded bloody fantastic. The painful sense of longing subsided with the fading memory of the good stuff. It was as if someone had eased off the pedals on my grief. I couldn't miss what I didn't know, or no longer remembered. This was yet another example of hanging in there long enough for time to remedy the situation while I sat back with popcorn.

Time did more than just help me forget. It helped me in other ways too.

In a functioning auditory system, the brain triangulates sounds coming in through both ears to locate their direction. This calculation happens lightning-fast. With a dead left ear, I initially perceived all sounds as coming from my right. Over time, however, my brain trained itself to consider context when hearing. It did this so well that I thought I had sound direction back. My audiologist assured me this was impossible. For example, when the television came on, my head turned towards it instinctively. I no longer defaulted to my right because context said it was improbable for Hollywood stars to be in my garden. My resourceful brain must have repurposed old pathways because the feeling was the same as having sound direction. That was, until my children asked me to play a game of hide and seek.

Jet and Jade were hiding somewhere in the house, giggling. They taunted me with a "Mummy, I'm here!" knowing I could not follow their cheeky voices to their location.

"All right, that's enough. Tell me about your day at school," I requested as I wandered from room to room, searching. We bonded through conversation during a game of hide and seek, as only our family could. Life was different, but still had its charms.

My tinnitus had improved by leaps and bounds compared to the start of the journey. After a year, the ringing had disappeared into the background, although forever present. I had learnt to ignore my screaming banshee, like factory workers learn to tune out the noisy machinery. I tamed my tinnitus by leaning into the experience. The ringing was all I could hear in my left ear. Without it, there would be a void. A deep, dark, and scary abyss. Absolute nothingness. I often sat listening to the screeching purposefully, with a twisted sense of gratitude. Unbeknownst to me, what I had done was habituate my condition. By leaning in to listen, my body learnt that this alarming siren was not a threat to my survival. Knowing it could not harm me, my focus shifted away from the tinnitus. I could finally brush aside the noisy machinery. Like a child that got ignored, my tinnitus dialled down its attention seeking behaviour altogether. There were times I could barely hear my banshee, even when I asked for her to scream to get away from the void. Sometimes, I even missed her.

On my unhappy anniversary, I showed up to my neurophysiotherapist appointment, ready to do more psychotic vertigo-triggering maneuvers. To my surprise, he said there would be no physical session today. He had admitted defeat and explained that we had been doing these same traumatising manoeuvres for a year now with no improvements. *No, no, no, don't say it.* He said it. He let me go. He officially released me from the hospital system with no link back to professional help.

"You have been with me since day one," I stuttered, struggling to get the words out. "I don't know what I'm going to do without you." I broke down, sobbing.

My health anniversary marked the right time to call it quits for him, but not for me.

"My neurophysiotherapist dumped me. He was just short of saying 'It's not you, it's me'. I am no longer with the hospital system," I ranted.

"About time. I didn't like having another man slam you down on a bed anyway," Tom joked.

I refused to resign myself to sleeping stiffly every night like a mummified corpse. Nor was I willing to be incapacitated by random episodes of vertigo. We have very little control over how our bodies run, as much of the administration work happens automatically. When our head turns, our eyes do not get left behind, fixated on whatever it was we were focused on. The eyes are programmed to track head movements with no conscious involvement on our part. During a vertigo attack, the mind perceives the world to be spinning. The eyes track the rapid spinning by darting from side to side manically. It would be fair for people unfamiliar with the concept of Nystagmus to believe they had witnessed a possession.

Tom would hold my hand and close his eyes through these episodes. It hurt him to witness his wife lose control over her body and mind.

I did my research and found a new neurophysiotherapist who came with promising reviews and credentials. It was a private practice, which meant I would have to pay for ongoing services. Being jobless, I preferred the free hospital system.

I walked into my first session with the new physiotherapist and felt disheartened when I saw a young man, half the age of my previous physiotherapist. If I couldn't be fixed by someone with double the experience, this was sure to be a waste of time. We spent the first session talking and laying out a plan. He thought it negligent for the hospital to administer the same treatment for a year with no discernible outcome. He promised that after six sessions, there would be improvements, or he would escalate the issue.

The physio introduced a myriad of new manoeuvres to steer my loose crystals back into place. None of these worked. He changed his hypothesis and concluded that my vertigo had nothing to do with these crystals. Rather, the vertigo was being generated centrally by my nervous system. I had been dizzy for so long that my nervous system could no longer interpret motion cues correctly. He requested I turn on my side to sleep and let the vertigo attack run its course. I then needed to fall asleep in that position.

"You have got to be kidding me?" I protested.

He insisted that the next night I was to repeat the process, but on the other side. I was to alternate sides each night until my next appointment with him.

I took over two hours to get to sleep on the first night. My heart pounded as I was flung around in my mind. Adrenaline surged through my body and remained in my system long after the spinning had subsided. My bedtime routine became snuggles and Netflix, hot chocolate, fluffy slippers, and then crippling anxiety from the scary vertigo that punctuated my nights. "Here we go again," I muttered under my breath as I lay down on my side for the sixteenth night in a row. I was being loaded into a fairground ride carriage that swayed on its hinges. I braced for the wild ride. The carriage rocked back and forth for several minutes before coming to a complete stop. The ride never took off. Well, this was new.

From that night on, I could sleep on my side, and violent vertigo was never triggered. I was still being rocked like an infant, but I could handle that. Maybe I could even learn to be comforted by it. The vertigo was gone. One morning, I woke up in a completely different position. I had fallen asleep on my left and arisen on my right to a pliable body. My joints didn't creak like an old treasure chest when I got out of bed. Blood flowed through my veins instead of cement. *Muah!* If I could kiss my subconscious, I would. It was permitting my muscles to move again during sleep. I hadn't slept properly like that for over a year.

I was excited to tell my neurophysiotherapist the great news. When I first walked into his office, I could not even look to my left without feeling nauseated and fearful. There are a handful of people in my life for whom I have enormous gratitude in my heart. These are the people I will never forget. My parents, without them I wouldn't be here; I owe them everything. The obstetrician who helped Tom and me to get pregnant and deliver both of our babies. Our children's nanny, who raised them during their defining years when we needed help the most. My bosses who bridged my financial gap when I got ill. And this young gentleman who returned my sleep.

"You are lucky I read a lot," my neurophysiotherapist said on hearing the good news.

There are two types of people in this world: those that can, and those that can't. Those that can, will find a way regardless. He found a way, showing up those with more experience, degrees, and titles. Getting ditched by the hospital system was the best thing to have happened, though it did not feel like it at the time. My regret was sticking too long with something that wasn't working. I shouldn't have waited to get dumped before I walked away.

My neurophysiotherapist referred me to see a neurologist in the hope they could treat the feelings of disequilibrium and head pressures that remained. He thought it was best to approach the problem from all sides.

The neurologist turned out to be the type that can't. She prescribed me a dirty drug that was used in the past to treat depression and anxiety. The industry had stopped employing this drug because it targeted multiple receptors and was messy. One fluke side effect of the drug was resolving dizziness in some patients. The other was a dry mouth. I had a desert growing in my mouth that turned my tongue into sandpaper and my teeth into chalk. I went back to the specialist to tell her that her prescription was not working.

"Double the dose," she said nonchalantly, "and keep taking it forever."

I was the type to take in sunshine and fresh water over *Panadol* for a headache. Doubling the dose at the flick of a dismissive hand did not sit well with me. I kept to my original dosage and continued to take the dirty drug, unsure what it was doing.

My healing progress plateaued after the first year. I was still experiencing constant dizziness, but it was tolerable. I concluded that I had reached the limits of my physical recovery and must live with the brokenness that remained. Time had done all it could, but there would be no complaints from me. I was barely noticing my tinnitus, had gained perceived sound direction, was sleeping well and the violent vertigo never paid another visit.

My anniversary marked the bend in the river of sorrow where the waters had slowed. It was my chance to scramble back to the banks and rebuild my shattered life. A person only had so much grief to grieve before the heart became saturated. The trick to dealing with trauma was to get it out in the open and then leave it behind. By whining, complaining, and speaking about my plight for a year, I felt heard, received the sympathy I needed, and gained a sounding board to make sense of the senseless. Trauma was an event locked in time, never changing in size or magnitude. I could, however, make the trauma appear smaller by growing a bigger life around it. The only way to do this was to seek new adventures, new experiences, and new connections with people. My trauma memory tile would be just one amongst the expansive wall of fresh memories waiting to be created. Organising chaos was my speciality, and I was keen to get started.

Chapter Fourteen

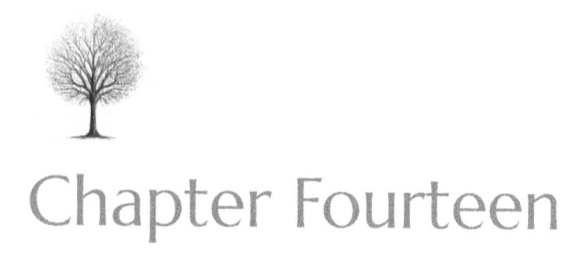

Gaining Momentum

A journey of a thousand miles begins with a single step.
—*Laozi, philosopher*

Our family took a drive south to Victor Harbour. We wanted to take the children on the famous horse-drawn tram to Granite Island to see little penguins. Jet and Jade rushed to the top deck, scoring front-row seats and panoramic views. The double-decker tram comfortably seated forty passengers and was pulled by a Clydesdale horse with adorable, hairy hooves. The horse snorted and clip-clopped, but the tram did not budge.

"Oh no! He won't make it, Mummy," said Jade, who we were starting to believe was an empath. I reassured her that the horse knew what it was doing. A few more snorts and the wheels rotated slowly. The clipping and clopping picked up speed. "He is pulling it so fast now," Jade said. "How is he doing that?"

Unsure of what a two-year-old could understand, I replied, "Momentum. You'll learn about it in school. There's no stopping him now."

I found that life, too, operated on the laws of momentum. The term "winning streak" and the phrase "When it rains, it pours" were coined through such observations. An injured fish doesn't get saved, it gets eaten. The rich get richer. Fortune and misfortune behave in the same way. A snowball rolls down a mountain, gaining momentum to become a massive force, either positive or negative. Before my tragedy, fortune favoured me well—it was celestial.

For forty years, I travelled through life without hitting a red light. I never experienced unrequited love, failure, rejection, bullying, nor made an enemy. Success came easily throughout my schooling. Every application I submitted—whether for scholarships, university placements, or job positions—was accepted. It was as if my dice were loaded. When I took up cooking as a hobby, I was selected out of thousands of applicants to compete on a prime-time cooking show on national television, despite having little culinary experience. So of course, I felt favoured by fate. The universe even gave me a sign when I met my husband-to-be.

Tom and I were on our first date. We stepped outside the German restaurant where we had dined and noticed a blue, shimmery rainbow stretching across the night sky. It wasn't the Northern Lights. We lived in South Australia, as far from the Aurora Borealis as geographically possible.

"This is crazy. Are you seeing this, or is it just me?"

"I can see it," I replied. I wanted to gauge other people's reactions but the streets were empty. This heavenly show was just for us.

"Aliens!" Tom exclaimed. It was his default explanation for paranormal activities in the sky. This light mesmerised us. We stood by the side of the road, taking it all in. Tom held me tight with first-date enthusiasm and perhaps to prevent himself from getting beamed up.

We were witnessing a moonbow. In the presence of a rare phenomenon, we both knew we had found a soulmate in each other. We spent our twenties gardening in the backyard until the wee hours of the morning instead of attending parties and clubs on the weekends. We cooked elaborate meals together and ate them amongst the hum of bees in our garden, admiring our work from the previous nights. If Eden was lost, we had found it. We were both old souls. He was me, and I was him. My life was a series of charmed events. The momentum was strong in this positive direction right up until the moment I got sick.

My illness was a force so powerful that forty years of positive momentum came to a screeching halt and then shot off in the opposite direction. Being deaf and dizzy snowballed into a loss of livelihood, profound isolation, and obliterated self-confidence and self-esteem. Inevitably, mental health issues ensued. The woe-ball continued to gain momentum. It was statistically difficult to have received the run of bad luck I did over the next two years. I couldn't have made this stuff up.

I would go on to experience crippling pain in the abdomen. An ultrasound confirmed that I had an eleven-centimetre cyst hanging from my almond-sized ovary. The weight of the growth had cut off the blood supply to my ovary, and my dying organ was the source of my pain. The gynaecologist suspected the cyst was cancerous and booked an emergency surgery to remove it. After a nerve-racking week of waiting for the results, the growth turned out to be benign endometriosis, rampant well beyond a cyst. It was a condition I would go on to manage.

My heart then gave out, jumping from resting to over two hundred beats per minute, and remained raised. Electrical circuits regulate the beating of the heart and mine had a short in it. I was left gasping for breath as if nearing the finishing line at an ultra marathon, only I was sitting on the couch all along. The paramedics reset my heart by administering adenosine intravenously. Bone-crunching pain spread throughout my body as the drug dispersed into my system, momentarily cutting all electrical circuits, and my heartbeat settled down instantly. After a few episodes of this sustained elevated heart rate, which I learnt was called supraventricular tachycardia (SVT), my cardiologist scheduled me for a cardiac ablation, a procedure to correct the abnormal circuits of the heart. Compared to Labyrinthitis, these health issues were an inconvenience at most because they were transitory. All I needed to do was wheel my vehicle into the body shop and drive it out fixed. Labyrinthitis continued to be my biggest challenge.

Misfortune loves company. I went out for a quick lunch and returned to find that someone had done a hit-and-run on my parked car in broad daylight. I'd parked my car in an affluent suburb and expected a note on the windscreen, taking responsibility. But there were no notes, there were no leads. Perhaps that was why these jerks were rich—they got other people to pay for their mistakes. I could understand accidents while driving, but to wreck my stationary car on a slow Tuesday afternoon was plain bad luck.

Had momentum been sustained in a fortuitous direction instead, I believed none of this madness would have happened. I didn't want to be the injured fish that got eaten. To course-correct the momentum that was heading straight for hell, I needed a sizable positive event. The problem was that all the heavy hitters were done. I have already graduated, fallen in love, got married, and met all the children I was going to have. Perhaps I could aggregate many small wins and their sum might prove adequate? Reversing the direction back to a good wicket was going to take a lot of snorting and clip-clopping. I needed inspiration to fuel my urge for action and sustain my motivation.

I came across the Roger Bannister effect. Doctors once believed that human physiology meant that man could not run a mile in under four minutes, as shown by the world record sitting stagnant at 4:01.4 for nine years. Finally, in 1954, Roger Bannister broke the four-minute mile mark. In the years to follow, this record would be broken time and time again by several runners. The psychological barrier had been lifted. What was once thought to be impossible was now demonstrated to be possible. If man could visualise it, then man could achieve it. I needed to know it was possible to free myself from the sadness of permanent and irreversible loss. I read memoirs of people that had befallen and got back up. Reading had always been for pleasure, but now I was reading for survival. I read obsessively, crunching through books like Pac-Man crunched through dots on the screen.

The Year of Magical Thinking by Joan Didion is a memoir describing the loss of her husband and daughter who passed away within two years of each other. Her narrative, though heartbreaking, was of solace to me because she made it through and continued to embrace the art that she loved, which was writing. In *Reason to Stay Alive*, Matt Haig explores how he battled severe depression to the point of an attempted suicide. He found his normality without the use of drugs, settling down to get married and raise a family. *When Breath Becomes Air* follows Paul Kalanithi, an Ivy League neurosurgeon who had to face his mortality after being diagnosed with terminal cancer. Upon receiving the grim prognosis, he and his wife tried for their first child together. He passed away with his daughter in his arms. He chose to live right until the last breath. *An Ordinary Day* by journalist Leigh Sales explores a myriad of case studies, including the Port Arthur massacre. In 1996, Martin Bryant gunned down and killed thirty-five people, twelve of them children. Walter Mikac lost his entire family that day: his wife Nanette, and two daughters, Alannah and Madeline. Twenty years later, Walter Mikac was still standing, describing his tragedy as a surgical scar, a wound that never fully healed but was possible to carry with him. Through these books, I rode on the shoulders of many giants, helping me to see the landscape more clearly.

I read many such books on personal tragedies turning to triumph, but one stood out more than the rest. In *The Diving-Bell and the Butterfly,* Jean Dominique Bauby tells of his abrupt transition from being a chief editor for *Elle* magazine to having locked-in syndrome. He went from a fine life to a confined life, following a stroke which paralysed his entire body, leaving one functioning left eye. That eye blinked out a sequence of alphabets, one by one, that became a bestselling book, published in multiple languages. While other authors tried to find eloquent words that described the resilience of the human spirit, Jean Dominique Bauby achieved this flawlessly and honestly through his delivery. I laughed throughout the entire book. In some parts, I laughed so hard I cried. It was an absurd reaction to a harrowing story. Here was a man suffering beyond comprehension, yet making a stand that his condition would not define or defeat him. The stroke took everything from him except his memories and imagination, and he used them to make his life bearable. If a man in that condition could make me laugh, there was hope. He fell from higher heights to lower depths than me. I could aspire to be a fraction of him. I found my inspiration. If he could, I could.

My motivation rose and crashed like blood sugar levels on a diet of empty carbohydrates. One moment I would feel alive and tackle the day with the ferocity of my former self, only to be held back the next moment by my broken body. I could not achieve results at the rate I aspired to, the same rate the previous me could accomplish. I had the spirit of a wild animal, pacing back and forth along the iron bars of my body's cage. The cadence of my need for action was inconsistent with the pace my body could keep up with. The frustration did little for my motivation, but somehow, I would find it again in this cycle of boom and bust. I needed to re-learn a healthier pace that was congruent with my current biology, so that "all or nothing" could become "one foot in front of the other". It is possible to move an entire mountain by removing small stones.

"I'm going to paint our house and sell it," I said.

"You know you can't do that anymore," Tom replied, looking worried. I had painted our entire house before with little trouble.

"Why 'anymore'? There is no before Nin and no after Nin. There is just Nin that this thing happened to. Just say 'You can't do that. It's too much work.' Don't say 'anymore,'" I said. There was a pause while Tom looked pensive, then his furrowed brows unravelled.

"I understand," he said.

From that moment, the split timeline of my life merged back into a continuous one. With those two words, "I understand," he moved on with me. I no longer compared myself to the previous Nin, nor did I keep measuring up to her. I only cared about where I was now, and where

I wanted to be, not where the former me wanted to be. Where I aspired to be was in a bigger house and not have my children believe it was the norm for families to eat dinner sitting on the ground around a coffee table. We had converted our dining room into Jet's bedroom. We couldn't squeeze any more efficiencies from our tiny space.

"Sell the house and move to where?" Tom asked.

"What if we found somewhere that backed onto a reserve? We can open our back gate and be amongst nature that we don't need to take care of," I said. Tom wasn't convinced, still mourning the lost dream of fishing from his own dam.

Each day, my health allowed me to paint a door or a wall before stopping. I would glad-wrap the brushes and trays instead of washing them out at the end of each session, since I made such little progress that more paint would have gone down the drain than on the walls. *Just keep swimming. Just keep swimming* replayed in my mind. The children had been watching *Finding Nemo*, and Dory was onto something. After a couple of months, our house was sparkling white, ready to be sold. It was time to look for a new home.

We spent our next three weekends at open inspections from the beaches to the hills, and did not see eye to eye on any property. We were embarrassed parents whose high-energy children terrorised homes at these open inspections. At one point, Jet and Jade had to be removed from dancing on top of someone's dining table.

"Let's skip open inspections this weekend and find a walking trail instead," Tom said, exhausted. Nature always rejuvenated our family. We could disappear into a forest and never return if we knew how to survive it. But since two white-collar workers would last less than twenty-four hours in the wilderness, we visited often instead. We searched on Google Maps for random splotches of green and headed out to see the real thing. We arrived at an expansive and immaculate parkland, more wondrous than all we had seen before. Ancient gums shaded the concrete walking trails below. The trails were dotted with canopied BBQ areas and small outdoor gyms. *Jet and Jade could celebrate many birthdays here*, I thought. There was a large flowing body of water cutting through the parklands that Tom made a beeline for.

"Do you think there are fish in there?" Tom asked, eyes lighting up.

"Oh honey, I could put up a picnic right here and you could fish all day," I said. Kookaburras sang their songs and fluffy ducklings waddled behind their mothers. Our children were sword-fighting with sticks, picking up ever bigger ones as they found them. In that moment, we found ourselves standing back on the hill of the twenty-acre property, hand in hand, dreaming. We spent the day lost in this magnificent parkland that had been mowed and kept on our behalf.

"The sun is setting. We'd better head home," Tom said. No one wanted to. We reluctantly piled into the car and started back.

"Stop!" I shouted, pointing to an open inspection sign.

The open house was about two blocks away from the parkland where we had spent the day; not backing onto it, but a just short stroll would get us back to Narnia. There was a commotion short of putting on a sausage sizzle. The turnout of people was greater than the combined crowd at three weeks' worth of previous inspections we had attended. The house looked ordinary from the outside, a heritage home with a cream sandstone facade. I was keen to find out what the fuss was about.

As soon as I stepped into the house, I was greeted with a corridor so wide that my outstretched arms could not touch the walls. The corridor was more like a grand hall, adorned with four dripping chandeliers, that opened to a living area fit to hold a ball. The space kept expanding as we advanced to a decked entertainment area installed with outdoor heating, fans, a wood-fired pizza oven, a fridge, and a BBQ. It overlooked a lap pool and a granny flat. My ageing mum could come and live with us. Dad had remarried, and it was too awkward to take them on too. There could only be one queen bee in the hive, and that was my mother. Tom knew from the look on my face that we would grow old together in this house.

The auction was in two days and the price was three times that of our current home. That was the price we had to pay for our children to grow up in a graffiti-free suburb, with no upturned trolleys and torched cars. I had squirrelled away plenty of nuts for a rainy day, at the expense of an expensive lifestyle. We had been living well below our means for far too long. Tom never understood why we needed a substantial just-in-case fund, but my risk-averse nature could not sleep without it. Everything was overdue for an upgrade, but I kept squirrelling nuts. The neighbourhood knew when Tom returned home from work by the high-pitched screeching his car made. That was my cue to unlock the front door because "Daddy's home, kids."

"We need to make this happen," I pleaded.

"Can we afford it?" Tom asked.

"We will need to use our savings."

"The auction is in two days," Tom said.

"Organising is my speciality. Negotiating is yours. You do your bit and I'll do mine." I began biting my nails. "We'll just have less rainy-day fund."

"It's already rained, darling. It's raining right now for our family. This is what you have been saving for."

Tom was right. Life was fickle. No one could guarantee tomorrow. A healthy body could break overnight; I knew that now. My financial strategy for our family based on our immortality, which looked decades into the future, needed to change. The promise of living to ninety years old was an illusion, a gamble at best. It was time Tom drank fine scotches, and I raised our children in our dream home. It was time to create new memories.

We agreed that Tom would attend the auction after work while I took the children to swimming lessons. Based on the enormous crowd at the inspection, our chances of winning the house were slim. There was no point in both of us being there for an unlikely outcome.

That night, Tom waltzed through the door with a bottle of champagne and a bound folder. He tossed them both on the bed, freeing his arms for a celebratory embrace. I grinned, knowing full well what had happened.

"The house is ours, baby," Tom announced, officiating the news.

I smiled throughout Tom's tall tale of the auction. He told it like a pirate who had just docked after a long voyage. The fight was down to him and another gentleman, an overseas investor from China, who seemed to have unlimited money. In the end, Tom's negotiation skills prevailed, closing the deal at under our agreed price, and significantly under the seller's reserve price. Together, we had formed a positive snowball, or so we thought.

We engaged a builder to fix up our house before moving in. I had a conversation with him in the privacy of our backyard and asked him to send through the invoice for a precise sum we had negotiated. I received the invoice by e-mail as expected. The content contained the summary of our conversation privy to only me and the builder. The invoice was on a familiar letterhead I had received before, to the exact sum that was agreed upon. There was no reason to suspect fraudulence. I paid it. The builder never received it. A scammer had intercepted our e-mail and kept everything the same except the bank account details where I had deposited six thousand dollars. We couldn't recover the money, so I had to pay the builder again. "Just teething pains love, we'll move in soon enough," Tom said. Misfortune had followed us to our new address.

Once the renovations were completed, we moved in and breathed a sigh of relief. The fresh paint and carpets smelt inviting.

On the second night in our new home, I was overwhelmed by an overpowering stench. I wandered around the house to find the source of the smell and stepped barefoot into our flooded corridor. When I flicked on the lights, I realised I was ankle-deep in sewage. I got acquainted with my neighbour's mess before meeting them. A blockage on the main road had caused sewage to overflow into our house from every drain. That's three bathrooms and a laundry. I did not want to traipse my soiled feet back into the clean living room and had to wade through the muck until I reached the backdoor. The corridor felt like it stretched for miles.

"Tom, bring the disinfectant!" I screamed. He got up from the couch and headed for the corridor.

"Don't use the corridor!"

I could not bring myself to touch my own feet for the next three months, regardless of how hard I scrubbed. If I could detach my feet from my body, I would have. The utility company rectified the situation and informed me that this was the first escape liquid incident in the history of this house. Two days in a heritage home that had been standing for hundreds of years and it had to happen to us on our second night there? The new paint and carpets didn't smell fresh anymore.

My analytical mind was convinced that this amount of bad luck defied the odds. At first glance, there was no iota of a thread connecting these misfortunes, but somehow, they congregated in clusters. There had to be an explanation that tied it all together. What if I had never got ill, and Labyrinthitis did not happen? I would have been working on a Tuesday afternoon, eating lunch at the onsite cafeteria, not having lunch out. I would have parked my car in the secure car park at work, surrounded by security cameras, making a hit-and-run impossible. The builder would have sent their invoice to my work e-mail address, protected by an impenetrable firewall of the defence industry. No scam artist could have cheated me out of six thousand dollars. Tom and I would have moved into our twenty-acre hobby farm far away, as planned. We would have had no neighbours and therefore none of their sewage. My obstetrician delivered Jade via a caesarean just a few years before the discovery of my ovarian cyst and rampant endometriosis. After peering inside, he reported everything to be in working order. There were no signs of a cyst. Several studies have associated high levels of stress with increased endometriosis growth. Had my illness not plummeted me into the depths of despair and stress, endometriosis might never have grown. The brochure that came with the drugs I was taking daily for my dizziness detailed an elaborate list of side effects that included abnormal beating of the heart. I had been with this heart since birth with no issues until now.

It was all a little suspect.

Despite the false start to moving in, our family was grateful to finally be in our new home with more space. However, Jet and Jade's school was now thirty minutes away. Drop-offs and pickups were adding two hours to my day. I began researching schools in the area and was delighted to find a co-educational school less than a two-minute drive away. Jet and Jade could attend together. It elated me to learn that this school achieved a rating of 99.9 per cent. That was on par with the elite private school we had sent Jet to for sixteen thousand dollars a year. I was balled-over ecstatic when they informed me that the school was a public school and the education was free. The money previously spent on education could go to service our home loan. Things were working themselves out. The snowball we had been compacting in our hands was rolled and gaining momentum in a positive direction. Happiness was building up collateral again to offset the pain experienced over the last years.

The glimmer of hope came just in time—finding our new home and stumbling upon the children's new school. Tom and I were exhausted from the vines of misfortune constricting our family, choking the joy out of our lives.

You cannot win a battle with broken soldiers. When I got parachuted into problematic projects, the first issue I addressed was the team's morale. The first sign that a project is derailing isn't a slipped schedule or customer complaints. Rather, it's the rising internal conflict within the team, people feeling defeated at the pile of mess they are sitting in and looking for causality in their colleagues. I don't spend any energy resolving these conflicts: it's a trap. I resolve them by putting wins on the board as soon as possible. In an environment where everyone feels like they are winning, there is no fuel for conflict. Within my first week stationed with a business in chaos, I would assign a couple of low-hanging fruits for people to pick. These are the tasks that make a tangible difference to the success of the project but are easy to complete, taking only a couple of days to do. When someone finishes the task, they get to add a big juicy tick to a visual progress board. When generating momentum, pick the low-hanging fruits first. Let Adam and Eve get a taste of the apple. They will want more of it.

Tom and I were weary soldiers, needing to sink our teeth back into the juicy apple of life.

Chapter Fifteen

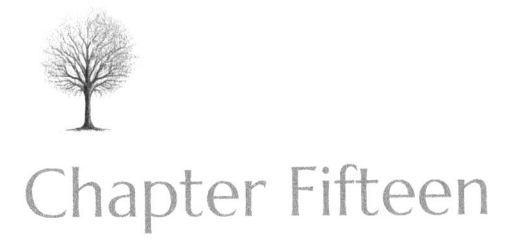

Pain to Purpose

Happiness is a butterfly, which when pursued, is always just beyond your grasp, but which, if you will sit down quietly, may alight upon you.
—*Nathaniel Hawthorne, novelist and short story writer*

Despite being a bright and cheery day, sunlight barely reached the ground of the forest. Dense plant life and canopies of giant trees shielded it from the rays. Weaving in and out through the thick, tall trunks was a colourful little parrot. He enjoyed berries all day long at the rate his eyes spotted them. His waste, full of seeds, would drop onto the ground as he flitted along his path. The seeds sprouted, growing into trees wherever he flew and re-populating the lush green lungs of the Earth. Oxygen levels rose, saturating the atmosphere, and all living creatures breathed effortlessly that night.

Every day was the same. The little parrot grew restless with his routine; there had to be more to life than this. The parrot began questioning his existence. Was he destined to fly as high as he could go? Or was he meant to build an impressive and enviable nest? Perhaps he was to preen his feathers tirelessly in pursuit of the fairest status. Plagued by the pressures of making the right decision, the little parrot finally settled on a noble mission. He was to build a nest he would be proud to call home. After all, he had a natural talent for weaving twigs, and by doing so, he would produce something useful. He was passionate about getting started. It all felt very right.

The next day, the little parrot knuckled down from dawn to dusk, building his forever nest diligently. His feathers became ruffled and dusty, a small price to pay for the long, laborious days. He barely ate any berries. He barely excreted any seeds. The few seeds he did produce, he scattered near his nesting site. These seeds sprouted into seedlings that struggled to grow, crammed on top of one another. Many did not survive, and hardly any matured into trees.

Long after he finished building his nest, the little parrot never again flew freely through the forest, nor did he enjoy the smorgasbord of flavourful berries he used to love. Instead, he stayed in his nest, savouring his accomplishments. He'd invested all he had into this project, and he was going to make the most of it. Cosy in his nest, the little parrot beamed with pride that he'd had a vision of his purpose and worked tirelessly to see his idea come to fruition. With his beak and wings, he had built a grand nest to perfection.

That night, however, the lungs of the Earth wheezed a little, and the animals of the kingdom worked harder to draw their breath. Little did the parrot know that simply by existing, he could do more good than he understood. His existence provided shade, many homes, and air that was essential to life on Earth. His existence was enough.

I wrote this short story to give myself permission to breathe and just be. To remind myself that I did not need to accomplish significant feats for my life to feel worthwhile.

Raising children to become model adults was such a long game that the days blurred into monotony. I easily lost sight of the direction I was heading and what my contributions were. As an avid gardener, I knew that weeds eventually overran any unproductive land, and I was drifting aimlessly. I needed something else to fill the void left by my career, something interesting, worthwhile, and more suitable for me. Not knowing which path to take would be unsettling enough, only I could not see any paths at all.

I had half a map to traverse the terrains of life but could not grasp the full picture. Society had taught me how to build a life, but not how to wind it down. Winding down usually happened at the end of life, but it was not uncommon for it to occur earlier, like in my case. I was never taught how to taper off gracefully. I missed being at work and having a sense of purpose. I missed the hunt, knowing I contributed to putting food on the table. I missed experiencing the feeling of elation when I achieved a goal. Without knowing how to wind down, there was angst in my heart to continue striving at a pace my body could not sustain. I needed to quell that angst before it could blossom into disappointment and then into depression.

Subliminal messaging to be successful is ever present, and society has a very precise definition of it. My parents raised me to the best of their abilities. They instilled drive, determination, and diligence in me to succeed so that I could lead a more comfortable life than they did. They didn't want to see me struggle and believed the next generation should outshine the last. Well-intended teachers did the same. They told us we could reach for the stars and become anything we aspired to be. They encouraged us to work hard for our dreams and to get back up after each failure. The script given to me was to get a good education, a good job and to raise a family. This strategy was decent, and I was happy with where I had ended up because of it. My work used the same script. It rewarded people for achieving outcomes that contributed to the bottom line of the organisation: delivering goals that customers would pay for, increasing productivity through efficiency gains, and motivating and developing people. Society had defined what it meant to be a success, and I used to fit that definition like a lock and key. They rewarded me for fitting in, and I loved the feeling. Now my bent keys were not opening doors, and I needed a new mental model to cope, or at least the other half of the map.

I thought of the parable of the monk and his raft. A monk built a raft to cross a stream, to get away from imminent danger. Upon reaching the other side, he felt gratitude for the raft that had saved his life and could not part with it. He carried the raft on his back, trekking through the dense forest. The cumbersome raft hit trees as he went. What once saved his life had become a burden. He lay it down and walked away, acknowledging that it had served its purpose. The raft was my career. Jade's vulnerable health once pleaded for me to put down my raft. There were several instances where we had to call an ambulance because Jade's asthma had become out of control and I was stuck in a meeting. Yet, I continued to carry the raft. Now my own body was asking for my faithfulness. What I didn't do for my daughter, could I finally do for myself? For us? I acknowledged that my work had bought my first car and paid for our wedding. It had bought us a wonderful new home to raise our growing family. But I was in a different place now. It was time I laid down my career, and I did so with an overwhelming sense of gratitude.

I continued to find novel ways to reassure myself that it was acceptable to sit idle while I did not have the answers.

Laying debilitated and ill delivered another unabridged truth. The finitude of my time was real. Knowing in theory that death eventually comes doesn't hit home the same way as knowing it through lived experiences. Four decades ago, I emerged from the darkness and into the light. Soon I would have to return to the eternal darkness from which I came. This realisation made me appreciate that my brief time in the sun was both special and insignificant all the same. It is okay to make something of it, and it is also okay not to. I understood that I was inconsequential and everything I amassed was therefore also inconsequential. A couple of centuries from now, my cherished car will be rusting in landfills. Another family will occupy the home that we worked hard to upkeep. They will create their memories and ours will fade. The march of progress will supersede my work and creations. What once was my fact will become fiction. There were no catastrophic consequences to my idleness.

Yet, I continued to be polarised and preoccupied by the dichotomy mindset that was bombarding me. On the one hand, there was the 10X script, as set out in Grant Cardone's book, *The 10X Rule*. The 10X mindset is about having it all and doing whatever it takes to achieve it. It urged me to push against all odds and continue to make something of myself, regardless. Then there was The Minimalist Camp, which rebelled against the 10X script. The Minimalist mindset is about paring down possession and busyness, stripping back to the essentials of what is important, which are relationships and free time. It coaxed me to slow down, to reduce the wear and tear on my body and mind. Minimalism was the permission I needed to aspire to less, to live simply, which was highly convincing because conventional success was becoming too difficult and out of reach.

I would have loved to embrace minimalism with both arms, but ultimately, I could not find my truth in it. This path of least resistance felt contrived. The Minimalist founders have spread their word through podcasts, *Netflix* shows, books, and world tours. They have amassed millions of followers across their social media platforms, which takes a huge amount of effort to maintain. Minimalism is being delivered in a 10X way! The human spirit, it appears, wants to strive and thrive to the level that it can. Perhaps we aren't meant to wind down. Perhaps we should keep building a life right up to the day we die.

When I compare the brief span of my life against the timeline of the Universe, the pace seems irrelevant. It matters not whether I am sprinting or crawling through the infinitesimal slot allocated to me. Power isn't in pace. Power is in purpose. The Business Improvement Department at work had a saying, "Efficiency can take you down the wrong path faster." It is the direction that matters, not the gears. Idleness provided the space to think and pivot my direction. I wasn't idle: I was thinking. No weeds would grow here.

Seneca, a Roman philosopher, is attributed to have said, "If one does not know to which port one is sailing, no wind is favourable." I humbly disagree. I knew exactly what port I was heading for and was travelling well in that direction. Then the wind changed. My firm belief in needing to achieve goals made me cling to old plans long after they were foiled. I grieved my potential that would go unrealised. The truth was, I wasn't the writer of my story. Fate simply included me in the plot. I mistook writing a few subplots as being the author of my destiny. Major life-changing events rarely happen according to plans. Falling in love with Tom or falling ill in my prime—I never aimed for those ports but docked there all the same. One was favourable, the other was not. Perhaps if I stopped directing and simply opened my mind, I would open all ports. If one does not know to which port one is sailing, all winds are favourable. My purposeless days became filled with exciting possibilities. When one is without purpose, the fun is in finding it.

"Mummy, would you rather be naked in public or have me die?" Jade asked.

"Sweetheart, I would rather be naked in the middle of Times Square than have you die." These were the questions small minds pondered, but they were significant. Jade was quantifying my love for her, which was as immeasurable as the ocean. I gave her a reassuring squeeze.

"Would you rather lose two arms or die, Mummy?" Jet asked, exploring the boundaries of what made life worthwhile enough to carry on.

"I would rather lose two arms," I replied, "because I still get to see you two every day."

"Same here," Jet said with eyes deep in thought. "Without arms, I won't be able to do a lot of things, but I could still do some things. I could eat ice cream and kick the footy. How would I eat the ice cream? Like a bird, I suppose. But dead, I can't do anything."

His resilient conclusion was uplifting. There were plenty of experiences to be had, making life incredibly meaningful. My career had bound me within a tiny four-walled cubicle for over two decades. I must be insane to want more of that in a hurry. Whilst the purpose of my life still eluded me, there were plenty of pleasures to be enjoyed in the meantime. Those pleasures that I had only felt apathy for since I became ill had a pulse again.

In seeking pleasure, I discovered I was not in love with my hearing. I was in love with life and all its wonderment. I was in love with music, bird songs, the happiness of my children expressed as laughter, vibrant busy cafes, and a game of Marco Polo in the dead of night. Similarly, I wasn't in love with my balance. I was in love with serene bike rides, diving into a pool on a hot day and flopping onto a plush couch. I loved tumbling around with Jade and blowing raspberries into her chubby creases. She would laugh so hard it morphed into a mimed cackle with squinted eyes. Adorable. That's what I had been grieving, the things I could no longer do, big and small. Now I had a budget of saying "Pardon?" twice because on the third, people said, "Never mind, it's not that important." The message that was meant for me would go forever unheard.

Focusing on a small portion of activities that I could no longer do had made me lose interest in a plethora of activities that were still accessible to me. Seeking a life of pleasure was the lowest form of purpose, according to positive psychology, but I had to start somewhere. We are not born knowing our purpose; we have to find it within ourselves and pull it out. I did it once before, I could do it again. Starting at the beginning, I reengaged with my interests by changing the questions I asked myself. Instead of asking what I aspired to be, I started asking what I wanted to do with each day.

I drew, painted, and started a vegetable garden at our new home. Our family drove to Lake Bumbunga, a couple of hours away. Tourists came from around the world to lay eyes on Australia's pink lake phenomenon. It had been on my bucket list, but work had always taken precedence.

"Everything is pink Ma Ma!" Jade screamed. She ran across the pink crystal sands and into the water, saturated with salt. Jet went exploring, picking up and examining crystallised flora and fauna. If Fairy Floss Land existed, we were standing in the middle of it.

Our family farm hopped; we spent our days picking strawberries, figs, apples, cherries, and sunflowers, depending on the season. Jet and Jade had never seen snow, so we drove for hours to experience it. At the first sign of white dusting on trees, the seatbelts got unbuckled, and no bottoms remained in their seats. Jade made it to the end of the toboggan run on her first go, beaming with pride. In her bulky winter gear, she was as wide as she was tall. I would have had to be a psychopath not to smile. Driving down from the snowcapped mountains, we found ourselves in a cloud, surrounded by thick haze.

"I have never breathed in a cloud before," exclaimed Jet.

I weighed up 0.2 grams of yeast on a microscale and learnt to knead a long ferment Napoli pizza dough, the kind where the puffy crust borders a paper-thin, crispy base. The precision required for a spectacular outcome was more science than art. Tom fired up our wood pizza oven, and we hosted a steady stream of family and friends who declared it to be the best pizza they had ever tasted.

"What's this weekend's adventure?" became the anticipated question for our family throughout the week.

"We are going to pick up some sugar gliders," I announced. The children shrieked with joy. We named our furry marsupials Blue and Brie, after our favourite cheeses.

Finding purpose through play, pleasure, and experiences had defibrillated my life back into being. This resulted in the happiest year of my life.

Chapter Sixteen

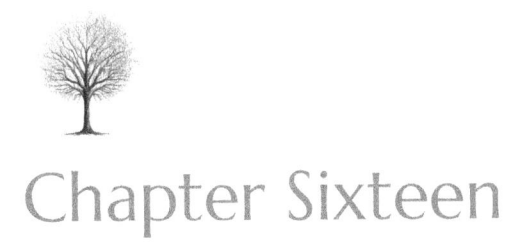

Search for Meaning

He who has a why can bear any how.
—*Friedrich Nietzsche, philosopher*

Anxiety and panic attacks were now mostly in the rear-view mirror. Now that I was in a better place, I was ready to dig deeper.

Viktor E. Frankl was a professor of neurology and psychiatry best known for his work in existential logotherapy. He developed a psychotherapeutic approach centred on finding meaning and purpose in life that, he claimed, fuelled the human spirit. In his book *Man's Search for Meaning*, he recounts an insightful story about a patient who lost his wife and was overwhelmed by grief. Frankle reframes his patient's perspective by asking, "If you had died first, what would it have been like for her?" His patient responded that it would have been incredibly difficult for her and that his wife would have fallen apart without him. Frankl pointed out that he had spared his wife this immense suffering by carrying the grief on her behalf. The man, though still sad, no longer felt powerless. He had found meaning in his suffering. He could carry the grief instead of his wife.

My illness forced me to slow down, something I needed but would never have done for myself. Being deaf and dizzy had graced me with the opportunity to get to know my children. I had even developed mounds of patience in the pursuit, a virtue I was previously lacking. My relationship with my children blossomed and became multifaceted. I was now their coach, cheer squad, and confidante. In the eighteen months that I have been nurturing them since my illness, my little ones have learnt to ride a bike, swim, cook, read, and write. They were even practising manners and consideration for others. I witnessed the magic of growing up unfold. Despite lacking a port, the wind blew me in this favourable direction. I stopped feeling like my children were hindering my career and progress: rather, they gave meaning to my suffering. With my children as my *why*, I could bear any *how*.

Our family decided that for one of our adventures, we would visit the place where we started our story together, our old home, now occupied by a new family. It filled us with excitement. The children were keen to jump back on their favourite flying fox and zip through the length of their old park nearby. Driving there felt odd, like I was in Shelbyville and not Springfield. The children sensed it too.

"Mummy, what happened to this place?" Jade asked the moment we pulled up to our former address.

"What do you mean?" I questioned.

"Our neighbour's windows are boarded up and there is graffiti everywhere. Whoever moved into our house ruined our neighbourhood. We shouldn't have moved away," Jet cried.

"This is what our suburb has always looked like, son; nothing has changed," I assured him.

"It never looked like this," Jet continued to protest, "this looks like the slums."

Our family loved our old house dearly and a part of us always will. As unfair to our old neighbourhood as it seemed, moving our family to an upgraded home allowed the children to draw an obvious comparison. They could not reconcile how a place that created their happiest memories now appeared derelict. The children's insight reminded me that love and memories would always be wherever my family was, no matter the postcode.

"You are right, son. Those pesky new owners destroyed our beautiful suburb. We shouldn't have moved away. Our poor neighbours," I said, preserving his happy childhood memories.

In hindsight, my tragedy allowed us to live a better life than ever before. It forced me to concentrate on my efforts at home instead of work. Order began forming around our family. Jade's asthma was under control, and she never took a ride in an ambulance again. We replaced Tom's car and could no longer hear him screeching from around the corner. It was a pleasant surprise when he walked through the door each evening. Jet never got into another fight at his new school.

"Hey Jet, why haven't I been called in by your teacher? Why aren't you getting into fights anymore?" I asked.

"At this school, the kids hit back," he replied.

For my children, public school was a better fit than the elite private school. The law of the jungle had sorted out his alleged neurological impulse control issues. My tragedy was not a waste. It had propelled our family upwards on a different trajectory. There was meaning in my suffering.

The sizable void was closing. Finding purpose in pleasure had brought me joyful anticipation. Finding meaning in my suffering had brought me contentment through the connection with my children. Dr Livingston wrote in his book, *Too Soon Old, Too Late Smart,* that there are three components to happiness: having something to do, having someone to love and having something to look forward to. I was missing the engagement piece, something I could sink my teeth into. I was missing something to do. Maintaining our home was not enough.

People randomly visiting our home would ask if we were expecting guests as they surveyed the shiny floors and cleared countertops. Our house ran like the Toyota manufacturing plant, built around Kaizen principles of continuous improvement. Systems were in place and workflows were optimised. The tea bags, teacups, and kettle were within arm's reach of one another for efficient beverage-making in the mornings. A visual inventory system ensured supplies never ran low. "I'm just ducking out for bread," was an unheard sentence in our home. House rules were outlined and upheld, even by the children. I did not permit shoes in the house, and showers occurred straight before bed, extending the time between cleaning the floors and sheets, reducing the workload. Our one-in-one-out regime ensured that clutter never piled up. If the children got a new toy, an older one needed to be donated. I arranged items in logical groupings. Allen keys got taped to the furniture they came with, waiting to serve their purpose instead of lying in a bottomless toolbox. Logistically, taking care of the house did not occupy all my time. I had capacity left over for another worthwhile endeavour.

As a manager, I'd been trained to match work with people's abilities to trigger a flow state which maximised productivity and, therefore, output. During flow, people are immersed in the task at hand, losing all track of time. The activity needed to be at the edge of a person's ability; challenging enough to engage and maintain their attention, yet familiar enough to not have them hit roadblocks at every turn, leaving them feeling deflated. Finding my flow was the last piece of my personal purpose puzzle.

A poster in the tearoom of the Information Management and Technology department at work described a Japanese concept called Ikigai, which translates to "Reason for being." The poster depicted four circles. They represented doing what you love, doing what the world needs, doing what you are good at, and doing what you can be paid for. The intersection of these circles was Ikigai, the activity that brings the utmost meaning to your life that you should be pursuing. While stirring my tea, I would examine this poster. I marvelled at how seamlessly psychology, philosophy, and logic all came together in that small diagram.

I would assess daily where I sat on the Ikigai chart. Doing what I was good at and what I could be paid for were the two constants that never changed. Their intersection was labelled as a "Profession," which seemed clinical and cold. Doing what I loved and doing what the world needed was a hit-and-miss, based on what was on my plate. When I got to pursue deep thinking work uninterrupted, such as complex planning or analysing a two-thousand-task schedule for correctness, inefficiencies, constraints, dependencies, and risks, I was doing what I loved. "Satisfaction, but feeling of uselessness," was the insight at the intersection of the pay, passion, and competency circles. This chart knew me better than myself. When I had to manage problematic people, perceptions, and politics, I would have rather stayed in bed. As for doing what the world needed, that was more contentious for me. I was a paper pusher, far removed from being a front-line worker who grew food, administered medicine, or taught the next generation how to read and write. Projects would get cancelled part way through due to budget cuts or direction changes, rendering the efforts of several months worthless. I wasn't convinced that I was doing what the world needed. Admittedly, a small void in my career had always existed. Ikigai was the holy grail, and I was at least close enough to bask in its glow.

Now that I was deaf and dizzy, working ten-hour days and attending back-to-back meetings was no longer ideal. An alternative Ikigai needed to be found. Anything that exists leaves behind a trace, like a strand of hair at a crime scene. Passion is no different. I started following the trail of breadcrumbs, hoping it would lead me to activities where I could achieve a flow state.

Could my love of good food be the solution? My parents practically raised me in their restaurant. After school, I would push the dining chairs together and nap until opening time. The tablecloth was my blanket. For every craving for wontons and spring rolls, I wrote up an order pretending it belonged to a customer and handed it to the kitchen. This environment cultivated my unstoppable passion for food: eating it, savouring the taste, and going back for more helpings. I would hold mouthfuls too long between chewing to extend the experience. After moving into my own place and having unlimited access to a kitchen, I discovered my love of cooking. I centred my days on meal preparation and eating. Sourcing quality produce became paramount. I wanted unlimited access to fresh herbs and vegetables and so I started a garden. My love of eating and cooking had realised my love of gardening. Passion catches on fire. One passion finds another which reveals itself.

Feeding the masses is a laborious job; I have seen this firsthand growing up in a restaurant. My parents had no holidays, I never got tucked in, and older siblings raised the younger ones. I couldn't pursue running a restaurant as my Ikigai. It suited my circumstances even less than returning to my former career. One day, I might find an alternative to running a restaurant to appease my love of food. Perhaps I could invent fusion small goods, a new genre of ingredients. Instead of fennel salami, I'd make coconut and coriander salami, the taste of Thai street food. Instead of olives marinated in Italian herbs, I would marinate them in Chinese chilli oil. Until then, onto the next breadcrumb we go.

I was a curious child with an insatiable appetite for learning and discovery. I recall an eventful knock at the door. My father opened it. It was a travelling salesperson. You hardly see them anymore. He was selling a set of Encyclopaedia Britannica. The internet wasn't invented yet, and my father said "Yes." They wheeled in several stacks of thick, beautifully bound books. I can still smell them. Between its hardcovers, I read about swans, rainforests, the three different states of water, and the solar system. I became addicted to reading non-fiction. Novels didn't exist in our house. My parents didn't know how to source the likes of Roald Dahl, Beatrix Potter, or Paul Jennings when they were struggling to speak English themselves. But they still wanted me to learn and did what they could.

I wrote down the facts I didn't want to forget. My dressing table drawer, instead of being full of lip gloss and bows like a typical tweener, was full of stationery—paper of all colours and thicknesses and writing pencils across all shades of darkness. These were my prized tools for learning. Facts extended to poems and clever quotes. I filled up books with insightful lines wherever I found them: in magazines, newspapers, or etched out on the back of the toilet door with the needle arm of a compass. My love of poetic prose turned into my love of rap music. I got into rap music because the lyrics were simply genius.

Work colleagues in their stiff suits would hop into my car for lunch, eyes widening when foul-mouthed rap blared. They tensed up as the bass beats vibrated through their bones.

"Can you please pass my sunnies from the glovebox?" I asked of my colleague in the passenger seat. He obliged, letting me concentrate on driving.

"Nin," he said followed by an apprehensive pause, "there is an envelope with a stack of hundred-dollar bills in here."

"Oh, I have to pay the electrician after work. He offered a discount if I paid in cash." I had just bought my first home and was preparing to leave the nest.

We had a short thirty minutes for lunch so I turned onto the main road like a getaway driver. An unmissable thump came from the boot.

"What the hell was that?" my colleague asked, startled, his body now pressed against the passenger door ready to roll out, depending on my answer. Between the gangster rap, the wad of cash, and the possible dead body in the boot, all trust had died.

"I borrowed my parent's vacuum to clean my new house. It has wheels." I laughed.

Rap was an unlikely choice in music for me when no one had ever heard me swear. I was the prudish adult that still referred to penises and vaginas as rude bits. My parents could not point me towards the Prep School reading list, so my love of literature found an unconventional muse in rap music. My absorption in word-rich tracks earned me perfect scores for High School English and the highest Grade Point Average (GPA) for my postgraduate thesis.

I was an immigrant, though. Immigrants can't earn a living by writing in English. Maths is a universal language. It was safer to become an engineer.

"I want to write a book," I said.

"Why not? You started writing one ten years ago," reminded Tom—another breadcrumb.

"But I'm not a writer."

"Start writing and then you are a writer."

"Don't I need a degree? A certificate?" I asked.

"Start writing!"

I started writing.

"Again, Mum? Late to pick us up from school again?" Jade demanded, crossing her arms.

"Mummy found her purpose," I replied.

"Everybody, my mummy is an author," Jade announced.

"Shhh, quickly, let's get out of here," I said, face reddening.

Winding down did not mean doing nothing. Winding down meant finding an alternative meaning within one's decreased capacity. In writing this memoir, I have found my flow.

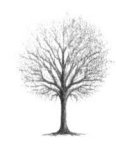

Chapter Seventeen

Powerful Perspectives

No pressure, no diamonds.
—*Thomas Carlyle, philosopher and historian*

I turned my Titanic away from the iceberg and set an alternative course. Momentum was being gained in the right direction. It was now about greasing the gears to make for a smooth journey.

"Darling, if you woke up to find you were suddenly my height and had my strength, would you be okay with it?" I asked.

"That depends. Do I have enough strength to kill myself?" Tom half-joked.

At just over six feet with a muscular frame, Tom could not visualise himself staring up at others and bringing the groceries inside one bag at a time instead of one car boot load at a time. He saw my smallness as a disability, whereas I have learnt to milk every goodness out of my stature.

"It's great being small. I can stand up straight in planes to stretch and my head doesn't even hit the cabin lights, while you look like a contortionist in a box; so uncomfortable." I laughed.

Being small made everything feel luxe: the house, car, and bed all felt bigger. The ceilings seemed higher. I was living in a castle while Tom was living in a house. To a great extent, disability is a matter of perspective. My children demonstrated that perfectly when they left the dinner table in the middle of their meal to spin around until they could not walk straight. They laughed and relished being dizzy, knocking into furniture.

"Mum, why do you complain about being dizzy? It's so fun," Jet said.

I had not learnt how to appreciate being dizzy, but I had enjoyed many serene mornings sleeping in, thanks to my dead ear facing the world while my hearing ear was buried in a pillow. Even Jet and Jade chasing each other up and down the corridor screaming couldn't wake me. There were many annoying sounds I could no longer hear well, sparing me from experiencing their full effect. Ruffling chip packets, lawnmowers, the top forty countdown playing on repeat in public, motorcycles, tantrums, and humble bragging, to name a few. Being deaf was becoming like being small; I was starting to see some advantages.

I thought back to being with Meena on the bus in Thailand and how far I had come from viewing disability with disgust to feeling sympathy, and then accepting it as normal. Helping a disabled person is still a must, but they ought to be helped like one would help a small person open a jar of pickles. From a place of equality, not pity. No one views someone who cannot open a jar with pity, as if their small size is a disadvantage in life. We should afford disabled people the same courtesy. I could now accept other people's disability with deep understanding. However, when it came to my own disability, there was still a way to go.

I hadn't fully accepted my disability, but I became content to be with it. Doctors reasoned that if I found acceptance of my situation, it would ease the mental anguish I was experiencing. But to me, acceptance was an impossible feat. The pressure to find acceptance and find it efficiently during those early days added to my stress. No one could accept a significantly worse life today than the one they had yesterday, especially when they were not responsible for causing any of it. "Change what you can change, ignore the rest," one of my bosses used to say. Acceptance isn't the delightful embrace of a short-changed situation, rather it is the ability to acknowledge it. Like a large tree in my path that I couldn't remove, I simply had to walk around it.

What started as me asking "Why me?" and "Why not someone else?" turned into "Why not me?" There are thirty trillion cells in the human body and all it takes is for one to turn cancerous. It is unbelievable that I don't have cancer. Previously, I bought into the big misconception that the chances of having an illness or disease were slim, and therefore did not apply to me. The chances are only low for any single condition, but when considering the many ways human physiology can break down, everyone is a statistic for something, eventually. The chances and severity increase with age.

By the time I turned forty, I had already lost four friends—two to suicide and two to cancer. It was arrogant of me to believe I was special enough to be spared and that these four people were simply unlucky. I didn't think their stories applied to me, not even as a lesson. I viewed my misfortune as a grave injustice when really, misfortune affects everyone fairly. It does not discriminate between the rich and the ragged, nor the wise and the witless. She is the dependable leveller who has brought down the powerful, the connected, the rich and the healthy. Even Steve Jobs, the inventor of the iPhone that has impacted over a billion lives, did not escape misfortune. He passed from pancreatic cancer at just fifty-six years old.

There is a famous story in Buddhism about a woman named Kisa Gotami who lost her only son. She could not understand why fate had singled her out. She was inconsolable to such an extent that the village believed she had lost her mind, along with her beloved son. Grief-ridden, she asked Buddha to bring him back. Buddha agreed to do so on the condition that she found the vital ingredient to make the cure: mustard seeds from a household that had never experienced the loss of a family member. She visited many homes seeking mustard seeds that complied with Buddha's condition. Every house she visited had felt the loss of a parent, spouse, sibling, or child. Unable to find the mustard seeds, she became enlightened to an undeniable truth, that mortality and misfortune are inescapable and that she must deal with her situation like everyone else. She was not special.

I too searched hard for reasons and any thin threads of logic for my story to make sense. But there was no logical progression to my story. I worked hard for decades to earn my bright future, which got extinguished in an instant by an outside force, not within my control. That didn't make any sense. In the senselessness, I have come to realise that misfortunes don't have a coherent narrative. They just are. Swimming with sharks and getting eaten isn't a misfortune—it is cause and effect. Misfortune differs from that. American television host and author Dennis Wholey said it best: "Expecting the world to treat you fairly because you are good is like expecting the bull not to charge because you are a vegetarian." I wish I had known earlier the true nature of misfortunes, that they operate on chance alone, not on who you are, where you have come from or where you are going. There is no cause to seek. Misfortune won't allow us to satisfy our simplistic view that cause and effect alone govern our outcomes. I was not in full control of my destiny. Even stating I had partial control would be generous. Life is arbitrarily complex, with millions of moving parts all interacting closely with one another in this petri dish called the Universe. Anything can happen. No one has tomorrow owed to them. I went from feeling unlucky that this happened to me to feeling lucky that *only* this happened to me.

The human psyche cannot deal well with randomness. As a species, we love predictability—to know where our next pay cheque is coming from and that our spouse will be there when we get home. The arbitrary nature of misfortunes was especially difficult for me to handle because being in Project Management, I had based my entire livelihood on planning and control. I believed I was in control of every facet of my life, an incorrect mental model. This mental model had to shift. I had to learn that I could still plan all that was within my control, but be open to working with the rest, rather than denying or fighting it.

Fighting the sealed circumstances that were imposed on me was useless. There seemed to be an unpredictable force shaping my life, one I couldn't understand or control. Decades of hard work could be wiped clean instantly by whims beyond my grasp. I desperately wanted to hear in stereo and feel my feet planted firmly on the ground again, but deaf and dizzy was how it was to be. I was behaving like a child, throwing tantrums to extend the inevitable bedtime instead of complying and learning to settle in without resistance, feel the soft blanket against my skin and dream sweet dreams. It was time I behaved like an adult, growing up to match what my tragedy was asking of me. There was no choice but to rise to the challenge. Who was I to protest the constraints decreed to me by life? Not only was it exhausting, but it was also futile.

I often reflect on myself before the tragedy. She wasn't a terrible person, just lacking in life experiences. I have since forgiven her. For not taking a step back from my career when my family needed me to, for not understanding that mental health issues were real, for being judgemental to unproductive people and unsympathetic to the struggles of others. For believing that my accomplishments were my doing alone, and for being too arrogant to accept help. I was the tough cookie who didn't understand that others crumbled until I crumbled myself.

Imagination and empathy are a poor substitute for actual experiences. When I became a parent, I felt suddenly relatable to an entire demographic of people who were parents. People who understood the sleepless nights for all their uglies beyond simply being tired. The mood swings, the thick head, operating on the verge of tears and wondering why one is not dead after remaining awake for days. Empathy alone will never pick up these nuances.

"Can you believe Nick is now in year six?" I asked, referring to the son of my close friend. "Next year he will be in high school. My friend cried at the uniform fitting."

"Why did she cry, Mummy?" Jade asked.

"Because she didn't have enough money to buy the uniforms," Jet replied.

"Try again, Jet," I said.

"Because she didn't like the look of the uniforms?"

"No, Jet. It's because her son is growing up, and she misses him as her little boy," I revealed.

Life experiences are the only qualified teachers to transform a person into someone who is easily relatable to a wide audience. Having experienced sinking to the lowest depths of despair, I could now relate to and understand people who had experienced grief. Eventually, that comprises everyone. My tragedy has smoothed out my character and rounded out my edges. My vibrancy has dimmed, tempered by my struggles, but it has allowed me to form deep connections with many others.

There was a period where I felt I could no longer be the best mum and wife to my family because I was not the best version of myself, and physically, I never could be again. I was unhealthy and sad, I lacked energy, and let's not forget I had almost accidentally fed my young to a canine. At first, I had only felt loss, but as time went on through the trials, I became a better mum than I ever was. I became a mum who was present and patient. This patience extended to Tom, affording him compassion and grace after a bad day at the office. After running the grief gauntlet and emerging on the other side battered and bruised but unbowed, I feel qualified to help my family tackle their adversities in the future. I showed resilience and by doing so, instilled the trait within my children.

They got to see their mum's character in action. They got to witness my ideas, drive, and tenacity come to fruition. These were the qualities that had propelled me previously in the workforce, but which, until now, my children had never seen. They saw me reading, learning, improving, building, and creating daily. They saw me becoming an author.

"Mum, humans can do anything," Jet stated, eyes wide with excitement at the possibilities.

"What do you mean?" I asked, wanting to hear more.

"Well, if I wanted to walk around the entire world, I could. It's going to take a long time, and I'll be exhausted, but I could do it. It's about packing a lot of water and food," Jet explained.

"Yes. Sure, son. There is the matter of the sea, but yes, humans can do anything," I reaffirmed.

"Like you. You wanted to paint the house and you just went and did it. Then you wanted to make pizza. And you did it. And now you are writing a book. How many words are you up to now?" Jet asked.

"Twelve thousand. Fifty thousand more to go," I answered.

After school, he would ask me for the word count. I wrote every day so as not to let him down.

Not once have I told him he could be anything he aspired to be. I showed him instead. Our children came to believe they were capable through osmosis. I hope that they will carry this unshakeable confidence forward throughout their lives.

I could now stand alongside other people as their equals once again. I had reclaimed my dwindled worth. In her book *Grit*, Angela Duckworth mentions that people are inclined to admire natural talent over hard work. I believe it is because we admire what is out of our reach. Everyone can work harder, but that kid from China, Yusheng Du, who solved the Rubik's cube at the world championships in three seconds, whoa! We know, deep down, no amount of hard work is going to get us there. We admire him for his unique wiring and his ability to do what we cannot.

"Hard work always beats talent, unless talent works hard," Tom would say. This was my opportunity to prove such worthiness. I could show that after being struck down by unimaginable tragedy, I could get back on my feet. We have all known people who have endured circumstances so bleak that we think "If that was me, I would not make it," and we admire them for it. Their ability to weather the storm many others can't is a testament to their capabilities, character and hence their worth. True status can only come from admirable capabilities, not logos on bags or clothing. I had weathered my storm and now I could stand proud and (metaphorically) tall. To pretend status does not matter would be to deny our primitive make-up and the truth.

Humans didn't rise to the top of the food chain because of our hearing and balance. If that were the case, bats would run the show and not be hidden in unsanitary proportions in dank caves. The leverage humans have is our brain, the source of our unchallengeable intellect that has enabled us to outwit and outdo all other living creatures on our planet. My brain was my worth and what a blessing it was to still have it intact.

My tragedy shed light on what was important and sieved away anything unwholesome, burdensome, or insincere. I spent a lot of time in waiting rooms and invented a game to pass the time. The aim was to guess correctly if the displayed plant was fake or real. The guessing part I could do discretely, but the confirmation part looked a tad insane. I went around patting and stroking leaves. After a while, to avoid people staring, I became great at spotting fake plants from afar. Their sturdy green stems, shiny glossy leaves absent of blemishes, and void of pest damage. There was no browning or ageing. The plant was suspended in timeless perfection. The tell of fake people was no different and I no longer had time for them.

It was easy to be friends with someone on the rise who was energetic and possessed a positive vibe. It was a lot harder to be friends with someone who was weepy and couldn't join in on the fun. Friendship means little when it is convenient. My tragedy provided me with a golden opportunity to sieve out the ride-and-die friends in my life from the just-for-fun folks.

My tragedy had a similar effect on my materialism. I recall the first twenty-four hours of being admitted to hospital as a chaotic blur. Oddly, I distinctly remember the television playing in the background amidst the wailing of patients. I had learnt to filter out advertisements as they bombarded my daily life, but they had my attention that night. There were talking meerkats selling insurance, a grown man in an unrecognisable colour-block superhero outfit peddling unsecured high-interest loans, and many happy catchy jingles to sell anything from boats to upcoming reality TV shows. I didn't need a boat. I needed to hear and move. Ridiculous ads upping the ante to push consumer demands seem extremely irrelevant when one is surrounded by suffering and death. Where I was, human needs were more basic, like having air in our lungs and blood in our veins. It was a revelation of how nonsensical society had become. I was part of it and did not mind until that point. Like a snake shedding their skin, I shed my materialism that night, after which I would buy only what made sense, and not because it was shiny, would impress others, or because I could.

Brosnan and de Waal conducted an experiment where they gave two capuchin monkeys food when they completed a simple task. Each time a monkey pressed a button or pulled a lever, they were rewarded with a slice of cucumber. Partway through the experiment, they gave one monkey a better reward, a grape instead of a cucumber, which is a preferable delicacy to capuchin monkeys. For the same tasks performed, the monkeys were rewarded unfairly. The monkey that continued to get the cucumber protested, refusing the cucumber and expressing frustrations. The experiment showed a concept known as inequity aversion, where feelings of dissatisfaction arise because of perceived unfairness. Humans naturally have an aversion to situations they perceive as unfair, such as when resources are unfairly distributed. It is thought to be part of our evolution.

I felt this unfairness because forty-year-olds should be conquering the world, realising their dreams, and raising families, not cooped up in the house sick. This sense of FOMO was present whenever I saw people travelling, attending concerts, and enjoying their experiences, because I wasn't enjoying mine.

Before my illness, I had never felt competitive or jealous. I was always happy for other people's successes, genuinely. No one perceived me as a threat and that formed the crux of my likeability.

"I agree, you were not jealous or competitive. You were worse," Tom said. "You felt you were above everyone and there was no competition because there was no one in your league." We both shared a laugh at my underdeveloped character.

Everything leading up to my illness had come with little effort. I could achieve and do as my heart desired. Now everyone was out of my league, and I felt the pangs of jealousy. It is a hard feeling to swallow. It was suffocating. I now have compassion for anyone who is feeling this way.

The Dalai Lama had a simple solution to this, which was to compare down instead of comparing up. He emphasised that comparing down will bypass our natural inclination to feel injustice. Instead, it makes us grateful for what we have, and feel empathy and compassion for those who have less.

I thought about my friend who passed away from cancer when his daughter was only a few months old, leaving his wife widowed in her early thirties. While it was happening, I cried a river. We were not close, but it was the saddest story I had come across. Then there was Johnny Ruffo, a contestant in the third season of *X-Factor Australia* that I backed while the show aired. He battled with cancer for several years before passing away in his late thirties. Standing on the precipice of fame and success, after just being propelled into the spotlight, his illness stepped in and denied him the opportunity he had worked hard for. Being permanently hearing and balance impaired seemed like a small price to pay for the luxury of living to see who my children will become.

"How can you read that stuff? It would depress the hell out of me," Tom said. Soon my friends were asking the same question. I was reading up on catastrophes and stories of misery and loss any chance I got. I appeared morbid.

"It is supposed to make me feel better and grateful that this is all I have to endure," I explained.

The Dalai Lama's approach was effective as a workaround. I felt grateful. However, I also filled my mind with miserable stories, training it to focus on suffering and sadness. It wasn't sustainable or ideal.

I was delighted to come across Matt Haig's perspective in *The Midnight Library*. His thinking changed my feelings about missing out on life. He explained that every person had access to the same spectrum of emotions regardless of what life they were living. Potential experiences were plentiful and no one could engage in all of them in a single lifetime. The good news is that we don't have to, as most experiences unlock this same set of emotions. For example, you do not need to fall in love with every person to know what love feels like. He referred to human emotions as universal currencies—happiness, love, excitement, pain and fear are accessible to everyone regardless of the life they lead. Though my life had changed significantly, I was not missing out on anything because I still had access to all my emotions. Engaging in human experiences can be distilled down to eliciting these feelings.

For the same commodity, which is happiness, I had been paying too much. My children felt the same joy running through our garden sprinklers on a hot summer's day as they would visiting Disneyland, some thirty hours away by flight. Every person, regardless of the situation, could experience the entire range of human emotions. Knowing this, my FOMO turned to satisfaction and my jealousy dissipated. My disability had grounded me and I was now paying less for my happiness. I have unlearned the need for extravagance in order to feel happy and am relearning how to enjoy the simple pleasures of life. I felt the same happiness eating a backyard BBQ or Wagyu in a fine restaurant. Every feeling was still accessible to me. I didn't need to compare down to feel at peace as nothing was truly lost to me. I stopped yearning for happiness constructs that were out of reach and was glad that I was no longer paying a fortune for the same commodity.

I still ask myself if I would give up all that I have learned, including the fortification of my character, in return for my health and vibrancy, to lead the life before my illness, earning and adventuring. This question is really asking two things. The first is whether it has all been worth it. I would say yes, it has been worth it to realise my capacity to endure and my capacity for compassion. I now know how far I could go. The second is asking whether I would rather take the blue pill or the red pill. Swallow the blue pill and I get to stay in the matrix, leading a life of comfortable illusion. Swallow the red pill and I must face the harsh realities outside of the matrix, forever fighting the machines.

Tom chose the red pill. I chose the blue. His strength of character is my anchor.

Only there is no choice of pills, there is only the red one. And you will be tapped on the shoulder when it's your time to swallow it.

Chapter Eighteen

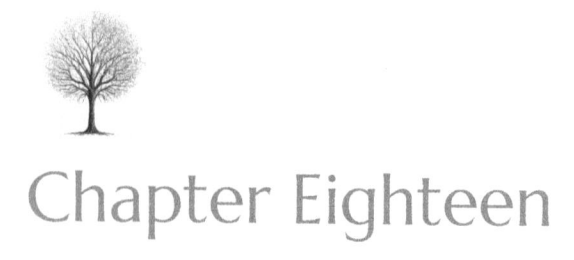

Acceptance

Acceptance of what has happened is the first step to overcoming the consequences of any misfortune.
—*William James, philosopher and psychologist*

I have come to recognize that the light at the end of the tunnel is not an exit, nor is it hope; rather, it is an approaching train that will run me over, again and again. An exit is what you aim for if your circumstances can change. Hope is a wonderful thing for terrible circumstances that might be fixable, where there could be a path out, no matter how narrow. But for predicaments like mine that are for keeps, that kind of hope only hinders and hurts. I had hoped that God would answer my prayers, time would heal my health, my resourcefulness be rewarded, positive thinking prevail, miracles granted (at least on Hallmark holidays) and lastly, I had hoped I was special. I could be the exception to the unfair, ugly rules in life's playbook. Hope held me captive in limbo between my imagination and reality, unable to move on. False hope, anyway.

I understood my diagnosis and prognosis the moment the doctors relayed it to me. I understood a phantom virus destroyed my hearing and balance organs and the effects were permanent. Comprehension was what I believed to be acceptance of my situation, and that occurred early on. I felt increasingly frustrated as people kept telling me I needed to accept what had happened to me. Did acceptance have a particular look? Were the edges of my lips not curled up enough? It took eighteen months for me to realise what they meant. Mentally, I had accepted the situation willingly, like an infant who accepts the embrace of its new stepmother. But my knowing soul and loyal heart were set in their ways and refused to welcome the intruding circumstances into my life. I already had a life I loved and was supposed to be leading. This wasn't it.

"With our own four hands we are going to build an extraordinary life for us. No plots, no plans, no man, no land is ever going to separate us." That was the promise I made to Tom on our wedding day. He slid the platinum ring onto my finger and locked in our vows. I was keeping my promise and we were on our way to extraordinary. Then BAM! I got railroaded off that trajectory to somewhere so different that even an ordinary life seemed unattainable. It took my heart and soul eighteen long months to catch up with my mind on the matter of acceptance, because acceptance was the toughest part of this ordeal. Acceptance that I wasn't just going through a tough time, a rough patch, but that this was it, this was my life forever. It turned out that genuine acceptance of a deplorable forever had a look after all. A look that only those in the know could recognise.

Tom and I were watching a documentary about shark attacks around the coast of Australia. For dramatic effect, the camera would start centred on the victim's face as they began their stories. Their physical scars, if any, were concealed from view. As their stories progressed, right before the plot reveal, the camera panned to the disfigurement caused by the ocean's apex predator. A missing limb, gruesome stitches up the torso and so on. Some stories were of near misses and the victims escaped with no horrid reminders except their memories.

"I can tell who has suffered permanent loss," I said during an opening scene. "Him. He has." Sure enough, the camera revealed a man sitting in a wheelchair without legs.

"He too has suffered permanent loss," I said. The camera zoomed out to a man with one arm.

"And he is completely over it," I said of the next man. The interviewee had gone diving as a group. A shark attacked a member of the diving party who did not survive his injuries (a valid excuse for not taking the interview himself). The interviewee did not sustain any physical damage. He lost a friend, and after a grieving period, his life returned to normal.

I could tell when a pair of eyes reflected my own. Eyes that were not focused on anything in particular, often lost, deep in thought. Eyes that were absent of childlike exuberance, because an inner child no longer lived in that adult body. Innocence had been robbed in exchange for knowing the truth, that the world was not all peaches and cream. The moment the victims became distracted from this truth, their struggles reminded them. Their disability, seen or felt, redirected their attention back to this truth. It was impossible to fully heal from a medical trauma that never stopped. Despite some of these cases dating as far back as thirty years, the heaviness in their souls remained, seeping through their gaze; the twinkle in their eyes tempered by realism and the weight of their experiences. It was the kind of heaviness born of relentless struggle that no amount of success or spring days can erase or make up for. They had, however, moved on with their lives. No longer stuck in limbo, waiting for their previous life to waltz back through the front door. Acceptance does not mean being fully healed. Rather, it means letting go of previous expectations.

I have learned to stop hoping for a light emitted by a choir of angels at the end of the tunnel signalling a miracle. The kind of hope I have now is in steady progress achieved through my consistent efforts, the wonder of tipping points, and the brilliance of science. A better possibility is waiting for me in the future.

I recall the story of the chained elephant told in a management training course I attended. It was common practice to cuff an elephant's ankle to a flimsy chain, pinning the other end into the dirt. That was all it took to stop a majestic and powerful creature from wandering off into the forest. The animal could easily uproot the restraint, but it didn't. The explanation was that they had chained the elephant when it was a calf, too small and weak to overthrow the setup, and so it stopped trying. As the calf grows to full maturity and strength, it never retests its change in stature and continues to be controlled by a thin chain. The key takeaway from my training was that we need to keep pushing the boundaries of what is possible because situations change.

My body was healing every day. What was not possible a year ago, or even a week ago, could be possible today. I needed to retest my boundaries, but it was easier said than done. There was still trauma stored away that prevented explorative behaviours. This wasn't simply a case of just do it. Legitimate fears held back horizon expansion. It was going to take consistent and considerable effort on my part to push through and break down those boundaries.

The story of the chained elephant delivered an encouraging message, but it was far from the truth. I was born in Thailand and immigrated to Australia as a child. I often visited my birthplace, home to these beautiful creatures. Many times, I have interacted with them. Feeding them bunches of bananas, riding them across rivers to bathe them, and watching them paint a vase of flowers with their trunks. They didn't need a chain to stay put. They willingly did so because the trainers had broken their spirits, evidenced by their scars. These elephants are subjected to cruelty, both psychologically and physically, until they learn it is futile to fight or resist. Their learnt helplessness results from humans breaking their spirit. In the 1960s, Martin Seligman and Steven Maier formalised this concept in an experiment that examined the effects of uncontrollable and inescapable stressors on animals. They have extended their findings to human psychology.

Seligman and Maier divided dogs into two experimental groups. The first group had a warning light that an electrical shock was coming. They also had access to a lever they could pull to prevent the shocks from occurring. In this group, they afforded the dogs control over their fate. These dogs learned to pull the trigger when the light turned on, to avoid the shock.

The researchers shocked the second group of dogs randomly with no forewarning. These dogs had no means of escaping their torture. They learnt to accept their fate and stopped fighting their misfortune.

In the next phase of the experiment, the researchers provided both groups of dogs with an exit so that they could remove themselves from the area where the shocks were administered. The first group left the area to avoid the shocks. Many dogs in the second group exhibited a passive response, which Seligman and Maier called learned helplessness. They remained in the area and received repeated shocks. The researchers had to physically drag them out to unlearn this self-defeating behaviour. Their bodies and also their minds needed to feel and relearn how to take back control.

Based on how my trauma unfolded, I was in the second group of dogs. But instead of shocks, it was violent vertigo that forced me to lie helpless and scared, a captive tortured by the relentless sensations. I could not move, get under the sheets to keep warm or call the ambulance. My suffering persisted until I was rescued, but even after that, I continued to be a victim of learned helplessness. I had worked hard on how my mind responded to trauma, and now it was time to challenge my body. My mind wanted to push boundaries, but my body wouldn't move.

To unlearn helplessness, I had to drag my body out of the perceived danger and have it experience the solution, allowing it to relearn how to take back control.

I booked my family on a flight to Melbourne, the shortest plane route available. I would spend fifty minutes in the air, surrendering to the motions and turbulence of the skies with no turning back, locked in for the trip. Valium, check. Vomit bags, check. Nine hours of restful sleep the night before, check. I was ready to board the plane. It may seem counterintuitive, but we decided I was to sit with the children in the row of three and Tom would be on his own across the aisle. I was teetering on the verge of a panic attack and the children were a welcome distraction.

The engine roared as the plane taxied. I felt myself pulled into the chair by G-force as we accelerated and lifted off. I shut my eyes tightly and clenched my fists. Tom reached for my hand from across the aisle and held it until my eyes opened once again.

"Welcome back," he whispered, "are you ok?"

I lucked out with clear blue skies and still air for the entire journey. The panic attack never eventuated, and I felt no dizzier than I did on the ground. My body absorbed a myriad of cues on that flight. Stale air, bells dinging to request attendance, tight confinement, loud humming of engines, and being rocked about. I learned these cues were not a threat.

"You did it, Mummy. We can go anywhere now!" exclaimed Jade upon landing.

"Our family is opening up to the world again," I replied, smiling.

Talk therapy addresses the mental side of trauma, while drugs address the physical response of the body. For full trauma recovery, the body, mind, and soul need to be healed together. My trip to Melbourne was healing all three.

Ever since then, every day, I have been mindful to carry out small acts to feed my mind, body, and spirit. I acknowledge and give thanks to my body through healthy foods, movement, and adequate rest. I feed my mind by learning new skills, reading, and embarking on projects that give me a sense of purpose. I uplift my spirit by being amongst nature, seeking novel experiences, and surrounding myself with positivity and people I love. On busy days, nurturing all three could be as simple as getting fifteen minutes of sunshine to awaken my mind and spirit, and help my body heal and repair.

Medicine has its place, but no medicine can replace whole foods, sunshine, restful sleep, exercise, meaningful connections, nature and inner peace. For the first forty years of my life, I derived my inner peace from being at the top of my game. There was no feeling better than maintaining first place in the arena you were competing in. Through my experience with Labyrinthitis and what happened next in my life, I came to understand that the source of my inner peace was born out of naivety, not truth. No one remains at their peak forever, but we need inner peace throughout life.

My inner peace is now derived from doing the most important thing on any given day to the best of my ability. This way, I can be sure that I am living the life I am destined to live and not stubbornly charting my course. I was indoctrinated into having clear, defined goals and focusing all my efforts on achieving them. Goals are great, but without a thermostat to evaluate the changes in conditions, charging blindly towards a target is like driving a car with no brakes. Reckless. Had I been focusing on the most important thing, I would have quit my work when Jade began to exhibit a multitude of dire health concerns. I had my children in my late thirties, by which time we had saved enough to sustain a one-income family for a while. I didn't need to work, but kept working at a great expense to my family. I was not living my truth, rather I was living an arbitrary life I made up.

Adopting the mindset of doing the next important thing every day has highlighted that life unfolds differently for everyone. I have stopped comparing myself to others altogether because I realise there is no basis for comparison. The unique lives of people qualify everyone to write a riveting memoir. If I have done my best with the life I was given and stayed true to what happened to me, I am exactly where I ought to be. Peace of mind comes from knowing that I am not supposed to be anywhere else but here.

My daily small efforts towards nourishing my mind, body, and spirit continue to incrementally improve my overall health. If we continue on the same path long enough, we will reach a tipping point where phenomenal changes happen. We can observe this phenomenon in the natural world.

The gradual change in temperature over thousands of years resulted in a spectacular transformation of the Earth known as the Ice Age. At the start, the temperature change was barely noticeable. The slightly cooler summers failed to melt all the winter's ice before the next winter arrived. Then ice slowly built up over the years, reflecting the sun's heat out into space, further cooling the Earth. A tipping point was reached whereby there were no longer any summers.

I don't know when my tipping point will come when I get to enjoy full health again. Not all tipping points take millennia to eventuate like the Ice Age. I witness the wonders of tipping points every morning when I boil my kettle for a cup of tea. Heat is applied to water and for a while, the water gets hotter and hotter. But the trend does not continue. A tipping point occurs when water turns into steam, stabilising the temperature. The same wonder applies to healing. I know I will never recover my hearing, but I know that I can feel better than this. I could be less tired and dizzy.

Working in engineering, I have witnessed first-hand miraculous feats of science. Many years in aerospace, and I still marvel when I see a passenger plane weighing over forty thousand kilograms glide across the sky, being kept afloat by mere variations in air pressure. Science cannot solve my health problems right now, but perhaps in time, science will make that leap.

Modern medicine has come so far and continues to advance through further research. There is research in the pipeline that examines different methods from stem cell and gene therapy to innovative drugs that stimulate the regrowth of natural hearing nerves. Reversing deafness is not a bridge too far in the near future. I look forward to it.

Clinical psychology coined the term "denial" to describe the period where I felt most hopeful. Hopeful that normality would return. It seemed counterintuitive to me that hope of any kind could be bad. I felt irritated whenever people discouraged me from hoping. In retrospect, false hope was denial. Hoping for something that could never be hindered my acceptance of the situation.

The moment I declared I was writing a book, I knew my soul and heart had caught up with my mind. The thought of writing made me feel free, and bubbles and tingles rose within me like a can of coke that had been cracked open. I had left the waiting room through the side door and stepped out onto a different path. I've smashed the rear-view mirror and there is no turning back. There is no more polishing of my resume, waiting to resume where I left off. Freed from false hopes, I'm charging towards a realistic future with sensible hopes and dreams.

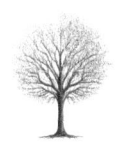

Chapter Nineteen

Parting Words

When you arise in the morning, think of what a precious privilege it is to be alive, to breathe, to think, to enjoy, to love.
—*Marcus Aurelius, Roman emperor and philosopher*

Dear Nin,

You don't know me, but I know you very well. In fact, I have known you your whole life. I was there when you were born, and I am here now, watching you become suddenly silent and still. I have been following your journey every step of the way.

I have watched you stitch your world together more coherently than most, a place for everything and everything in its place, both in your home and in your mind. Being healthy one day and debilitated the next is the ultimate disruption of order. It's going to be especially difficult for someone like you to process this senseless interruption. I am so sorry you are going through this. I know what it's like to be enjoying every facet of life and then, in an instant, enjoy none of it. Though it feels insurmountable and unbearable right now, if you give yourself some time, you will figure it out. I suppose you have no choice but to do so. Jet and Jade are still little, they need their mother. Your tragedy was not your fault, but overcoming it is your responsibility.

I imagine it to be as unfathomable for you as the sky falling down. Who knows, maybe that could happen next—after all, this did. Your claim on reality is shattered right now, but perhaps I can help?

I am a huge fan of the age-old adage, "A smooth sea never made a skilful sailor." If you are looking for a silver lining, this is it. It's not every day that you will face a challenge of this magnitude. Don't waste the opportunity. This adversity is the mirror on the wall. It will reveal deep secrets about yourself, both good and bad. I suggest you pay attention. There is no better time to improve yourself. These terrible feelings you harbour are the best catalysts for change. There is no greater motivator than wanting to put some distance between yourself and misery. Use the energy your adversity has afforded you to test new and better ways of being.

The sailor analogy aligns well with life in more ways than one. Set sail long enough and even the most skilful sailor will come into sizable rogue waves, a wall of water that he stands no chance of beating. There are immense forces operating outside our control, well beyond what we can conquer. That is not to say we are powerless, rather, we have to sail with the conditions to the best of our abilities. Fighting against the wind is exhausting and futile. To put it another way, life comes with a rhythm. You must dance to that rhythm, but you are in control of the choreography. Find the beat and step to it. Dancing out of rhythm looks absurd.

When you transitioned from engineering into management, your boss said to you, "What got you here won't get you there." He meant that when facing new challenges, you cannot repeat what you've been doing, even if it worked well for you in the past. You need to rise to the occasion through personal growth. In engineering, they rewarded you for being detail-orientated but in management, they penalised it and rewarded you for how well you summarised. Volunteering to take on more work yourself was no longer praised, but your ability to delegate to an ever-growing team was. To date, your can-do attitude and refusal to take no for an answer have served you well.

However, this problem you are facing is not created in a man-made world. Nature doesn't negotiate. You cannot work hard, innovate, invest, network, or negotiate your way out of this dilemma. There is no bargaining with a virus. If anything, the opposite skill is required; to be still and find contentment playing the hand you have been dealt.

This is not a tough time you can work through and have it checked off your list. It requires acceptance that you will never have the "good" life you planned. Knowing that your prognosis will never change is acceptance. You are suffering, but not because fate derailed you in a negative direction. You are suffering because you are fighting with fate instead of getting on with what it has assigned you. Without this acceptance, you cannot build an alternative future. You are stuck, living in your imagination, not reality. Sure, be hopeful of a brighter future. Be hopeful of advancements in medicine. But there is no hope of getting your hearing or balance back in any foreseeable future. That kind of hope only hurts, not heals. Acceptance feels terrible and it's the hardest part to overcome. You are going to have to eat this elephant one bite at a time. First, acknowledge that the next day will be the same. Then the next week and the months after that. When all hope is lost, you will break before you rebuild. Take care of your mental health.

Do you remember yourself in your mid-twenties? Jet-setting around the world on business class flights meeting with clients twice or thrice your age. You wanted it all, and it was within your sights, too. Only now it isn't. You promised your younger self a lot of things that you will not deliver on. Don't feel guilty. You owe her jack. She was healthy, energetic and starry-eyed. She passed none of that stamina and ignorance onto you. You and she are different people. You now know her kind of success comes with a cost to your health and family, a cost you are not willing to pay. With age, your mind grows wiser and your body more fragile. It's time to make new dreams and plans for the person you are today, the only person you are obligated to take care of.

Just don't spend too long making sense of the senseless. A virus goes where it wants to go. The world operates with millions of moving parts, all interacting with one another in a complex equation; it is impossible to untangle the what from the why. Don't spend energy looking for a logical explanation where none exists. When these questions creep into your mind, cast them out and carry on. Save your attention and energy for dealing with the actual situation. When bitten by a snake, don't analyse the situation and question why. Just deal with the poison.

I asked several of the people closest to us to describe the essence of who you are. None said, "When I think of Nin, I think of a hearing individual with acrobatic balance."

It's not just your body that has limitations. You also have self-limiting beliefs to address. You are not a lesser person because your body broke. These outdated perspectives need changing and that will not happen by thinking alone. It takes action. Results from actions inform your thoughts, and your thoughts dictate your next actions. That is growth. Sometimes learning means unlearning what you once knew. I implore you to challenge these self-limiting beliefs that no longer serve you.

Who you are is as vast as the ocean. Removing a tonne of water from the sea will not shake its ecosystem. Similarly, your health does not define you. You are more than your health, let alone your hearing and balance. You are a mum, wife, daughter, sister, friend, neighbour, creator, writer, visionary and philosopher. The truth can even stand on its own without these labels. Ditch the labels that make you feel small, not because of your prejudices, but because society is not ready to support them and therefore you. You are not defined by being disabled. Rather disability makes up just one of many experiences that pours water back into your ever-expanding ocean. This adversity will lead to newfound wisdom, loyal supporters, fortification of your character and will bring about exciting new endeavours. It's not all bad.

In a world that measures success by productivity, you are going to start off feeling inadequate in your new body, like you are getting left behind. You are not falling behind. To fall behind means there is someone else ahead of you on your path, and no one else is on your path. Your journey is unique because you and your experiences are unique. Only you are travelling on this path. No other person shares your predicament, innate talents, experiences, luck, knowledge, and resources. If there is a race, there is only one person in it: you. Run *your* best race and that's enough.

Remember the Thai proverb your Mum used to say? "Once ridden on a tiger's back, it is difficult to hop off." Your illness has forced you to dismount from your prestigious career, bruising your ego and self-worth. Your ego will fumble with the response when you are asked "What do you do for a living?" Take heart, a satisfying answer will emerge during your long walks in nature, while cooking a slow meal, or engaging in a joyful moment with your children. It is then you will realise that you now live for a living—an opportunity denied to many stuck in jobs while they would prefer to be elsewhere. Your ego is a made-up construct that you can change anytime.

When the ups and downs in your journey get overwhelming, try treating your emotions as you do the weather. Just like the weather, emotions come, and then they pass. Nothing lasts forever, good or bad. Yes, this gut-wrenching feeling included. Even the deadliest nuclear radiation half-lives over time and your turbulent feelings will too. Allow time to do its best work. Don't do anything stupid in a moment of weakness. Remember your purpose. Remember your family. My best advice to weather the storm is to be with it, sit with it and get to know it. You can't change your emotions just like you can't change the weather. When it rains, we don't try to stop it, deny it or label it. We simply work with it and work around it. You need to do the same with your emotions. Do not hurry them along, ignore them or suppress them. Acknowledge them and carry on. The worst thing that can happen to you is how you feel about it, and if you don't mind, then it doesn't matter.

Being denied the ability to move fluidly means you lost your right as a mum to tumble and wrestle with your toddler without a care in the world. Over time, she will grow up and you would have lost that right, anyway. However, that would be normal, not a tragedy. You are angry because you feel robbed. Only you haven't been. No one escapes misfortunes. It will come sooner or later and alter the course of perceived normalcy. Yours came now. This is your unique cross to bear, your story of suffering, enduring, and overcoming. Everyone has or will soon have one of these stories. You've never been one to shy away from responsibilities, so stand tall and carry your cross with pride.

Don't focus so much on your loss that you lose sight of what remains. You are sad because some activities and experiences that used to be available to you are now off-limits. Those privileges were darn amazing because life itself is amazing. It is wonderful to be alive. There are plenty more experiences waiting for you that are within your capabilities to enjoy. Get out there and reengage with the world even if you don't feel like it. Joy will eventually creep back in, and when it does, you will surprise yourself. The grief never lessens, but it can be made to feel smaller by growing a bigger life around it. Now and then, like an old book on the shelf, you might pull out your tragedy and revisit its pages. The feelings will flood back to remind you it never went away. All that happened was your book collection got bigger.

Little by little amounts to a lot. Saint Francis of Assisi once said, "Start by doing what's necessary; then do what's possible; and suddenly you are doing the impossible." Start small. Make your bed again. Wash the piled-up dishes. Pay the bills. Then, if you feel up to it, go for a walk around the block. Keep seeking pockets of joy in this saddened wasteland, and soon enough, you'll reach a tipping point where sunshine conquers the clouds. Finding an interest, no matter how small, to reengage with life is the beginning of healing. Passion, like fire, only needs to be lit. It will spread and grow on its own.

This adversity will become your armour. You will be stronger for it. Your hands are now up with your fingers spread, ready to catch the next curve ball that comes your way. You will be more ready than most to tackle life's difficulties and even the big questions—of your mortality and of those you love. This tragedy will give your life a story worth telling. You have lost your hearing and balance for now. In time, you will lose your entire body. And on that day, you can reflect and truly say you have led an interesting life of depth, worthy of capturing in the pages of a book, to be told and retold.

Yours sincerely,

Future you.

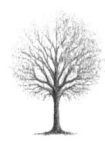

Leave a Review

> If you enjoyed *Suddenly Silent and Still*, will you please consider leaving a review on Amazon, Goodreads or your platform of choice? Not only do reviews help authors find more readers like you, but if you found the book helpful, others will too. I appreciate your kindness and taking the time to do so.

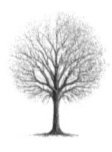

Acknowledgements

One o'clock in the morning, at dinner time, or during our small window of togetherness after the children have gone to bed, a thought would enter my mind and I would need to write it down. Tom never said a word. He let me be. He let me type away at my writing station, which started on one end of our dining table and expanded over time to consume most of the common area. Again, Tom said nothing. When I had writer's block, he lit scented candles, brewed warm beverages and upgraded my keyboard and mouse to entice me back to the craft. He encouraged me to write when I hadn't yet viewed myself as a writer. He was the first to read and review my manuscript, plucking up the courage to provide feedback, knowing I would challenge it because we were too close. Without him, this book would be an idea, nothing more. Thank you, Tom, my husband, my willing carer and my strength.

I give thanks to my father, a highly intelligent man who thought differently and taught me to do the same. He laid the foundations of success and resilience in all his children. He directed me to many leverages in everyday life that I use to my advantage. I recall him tipping the waiter the moment we sat down, explaining "Now watch him take care of us for the rest of our meal; there is no point tipping at the end." Thank you for your mind that I inherited and also for passing down your passion for reading and writing. He often said, "You are only as intelligent as your ability to articulate your ideas." He encouraged me to write. When I questioned what should I write about, he said "Anything and everything."

To my sweetest mother, who filled my heart with virtues true. Whenever we visited the local pond, I would feed adorable ducks along with everyone else. She stood off in the corner feeding pigeons and an assortment of other overlooked species. "They deserve to eat too," she told me. She is the rare gem that takes no credit for her efforts in the shadows. The maintainer of gardens long after others have claimed the glory of building them. I inherited my soul that points True North from her, which formed the perspectives contained in this book.

To my three sisters, who were there for me the moment I was born. Our family was dysfunctional, like every other, but I didn't know that. They all took hits so I could live in a bubble, never leaving an ideal world. I felt loved, spoiled, and cared for my whole life. Hand-me-downs skipped the chain and went straight to the youngest, me. I had more than I ever wanted. Even at the height of my career, they continued to pay for my meals when we dined out together like I was still a little girl. My strong sense of self-worth came from them.

Jet and Jade, my two reasons for being. I would climb Mount Everest if they were stranded up there. There is nothing I would not do for them, including getting back up from a defeat, and dusting myself off so I can continue to be their mum. They are the light in my life that shines on in the darkest hours. Without my children, I would have given up on life during its toughest times.

To Kunden at UpLit Press, thank you for believing in me—a first-time writer with no track record of writing. I am determined to be the right choice. It is easy to support people on their way up but to take a chance on an unknown at the starting line evokes unshakeable loyalty in my heart. Thank you for being the light, illuminating the confusing path to becoming published—a major bucket list item for me.

To my Beta Readers, Em Buckman, Elizabeth James and Kristina Gruell, three strangers who became my friends through their kindness. I posted up my first chapter in a writing forum for initial feedback, to determine whether I had what it takes to write this book. Three authors encouraged me to keep going and volunteered to read my raw manuscript when it was ready. Their early feedback was invaluable, injecting quality into my book that otherwise would not be there. It takes a village to publish a book, and they have become my tribe.

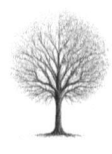

About the Author

Nin was born in Bangkok, Thailand and immigrated with her family to Darwin, Australia when she was a little girl. Darwin in the eighties was a big rural country town, not a thriving small city like it is today. She lived across the road from sprawling bushlands with a deep creek cutting across the landscape. After school, she would run into the wilderness with her friends and get lost in their sunburnt Narnia.

She lived with her family in the same apartment block as many First Nations people, who became her friends. Her vibrant childhood, full of simple country adventures, set the foundation for her values and who she became.

Nin moved to Adelaide, a larger city with more opportunities, to pursue her engineering degree. Teenage city girls were glamourous and wore blazers, and Nin did just enough to fit in. She graduated and got a job at a prestigious technology company. It was there she met her husband, Tom, while working on a fighter jet project. They moved mountains to be together and named their first son Jet to commemorate their story. Two years later, Jade was born and completed their family.

Her career followed a natural progression from engineering into management. She was working as a Project Management executive before stopping to tackle her trauma. With her newfound freedom, no longer shackled to the nine-to-five routine, she spends her days pursuing her passions. She loves to create, turning seeds into gardens, alphabets into stories, and ingredients into cuisine. Nin never dreamt of being a writer until the wind in her sails changed direction and gave her a compelling story to tell.

Contact the Author

suddenlysilentandstill.com
Instagram/suddenlysilentandstill

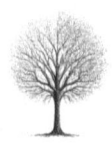

UpLitPress.co.uk

Publishing books that make you glad to be part of the human race.

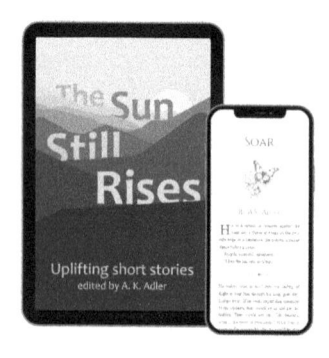

Get a free anthology when you join our mailing list

www.ingramcontent.com/pod-product-compliance
Ingram Content Group UK Ltd.
Pitfield, Milton Keynes, MK11 3LW, UK
UKHW031832170125
453762UK00001B/24

9 798227 221148